THE
EVERYTHING.
GUIDE TO
ALOE VERA FOR HEALTH

Dear Reader,

Do you feel like you need a little help with an aspect of your health? Whether you feel tired, anxious, out of shape, overweight, underweight, dehydrated, unable to sleep, or even depressed, there is a natural supplement that could change your life. This may sound like something that is "too good to be true," but it is supported by thousands of years of documented use. This supplement is not hard to find or expensive to purchase. In fact, it may be growing in your front yard right now. It's aloe vera!

This book will tell you the amazing things that aloe can do. You'll learn about its history, its healing components, and its beneficial qualities. From improving your quality of life to safeguarding your health, aloe vera has shown remarkable results in bettering many aspects of the body and its functioning.

Safe, natural, effective, and supported by thousands of years of use and modern studies, aloe vera is one of the most amazing natural remedies available to humankind, so why not find out for yourself what it can do for you? What do have you to lose?

Britt Brandon

Welcome to the EVERYTHING® Series!

These handy, accessible books give you all you need to tackle a difficult project, gain a new hobby, comprehend a fascinating topic, prepare for an exam, or even brush up on something you learned back in school but have since forgotten.

You can choose to read an Everything® book from cover to cover or just pick out the information you want from our four useful boxes: e-questions, e-facts, e-alerts, and e-ssentials. We give you everything you need to know on the subject, but throw in a lot of fun stuff along the way, too.

We now have more than 400 Everything® books in print, spanning such wide-ranging categories as weddings, pregnancy, cooking, music instruction, foreign language, crafts, pets, New Age, and so much more. When you're done reading them all, you can finally say you know Everything®!

QUESTION

Answers to common questions

FACT

Important snippets of information

ALERT

Urgent warnings

ESSENTIAL

Quick handy tips

PUBLISHER Karen Cooper

MANAGING EDITOR, EVERYTHING® SERIES Lisa Laing

COPY CHIEF Casey Ebert

ASSISTANT PRODUCTION EDITOR Alex Guarco

ACQUISITIONS EDITOR Lisa Laing

SENIOR DEVELOPMENT EDITOR Brett Palana-Shanahan

EVERYTHING® SERIES COVER DESIGNER Erin Alexander

Visit the entire Everything® series at *www.everything.com*

THE
EVERYTHING®
GUIDE TO
ALOE VERA FOR
HEALTH

Discover the natural healing power of aloe vera

Britt Brandon

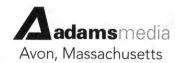

Adamsmedia

Avon, Massachusetts

An Everything® Series Book.
Everything® and everything.com® are registered trademarks of F+W Media, Inc.

Published by
Adams Media, a division of F+W Media, Inc.
57 Littlefield Street, Avon, MA 02322. U.S.A.
www.adamsmedia.com

Contains material adapted from *What Color Is Your Smoothie?* By Britt Brandon, copyright © 2012 by
F+W Media, Inc., ISBN 10: 1-4405-3616-3, ISBN 13: 978-1-4405-3616-8.

ISBN 10: 1-4405-8694-2
ISBN 13: 978-1-4405-8694-1
eISBN 10: 1-4405-8695-0
eISBN 13: 978-1-4405-8695-8

Printed in the United States of America.

10 9 8 7 6 5 4 3 2 1

This book is intended as general information only, and should not be used to diagnose or treat any health condition. In light of the complex, individual, and specific nature of health problems, this book is not intended to replace professional medical advice. The ideas, procedures, and suggestions in this book are intended to supplement, not replace, the advice of a trained medical professional. Consult your physician before adopting any of the suggestions in this book, as well as about any condition that may require diagnosis or medical attention. The author and publisher disclaim any liability arising directly or indirectly from the use of this book.

Many of the designations used by manufacturers and sellers to distinguish their products are claimed as trademarks. Where those designations appear in this book and F+W Media, Inc. was aware of a trademark claim, the designations have been printed with initial capital letters.

Cover image © fotyma/123RF.

This book is available at quantity discounts for bulk purchases.
For information, please call 1-800-289-0963.

This book is dedicated to my loving family—
my wonderful husband, Jimmy, and each of our
three amazing children: Lilly, Lonni, and JD!

Contents

Top 10 Things to Know about Aloe Vera

1. Aloe vera's effectiveness in regulating blood sugar levels and improving the body's ability to produce and utilize insulin is showing promise in the development of natural treatment methods for diabetes.

2. Providing antibacterial benefits, aloe vera has shown to improve the immune system's functioning and better the body's ability to fend off bacterial infections.

3. Applied topically to wounds on the skin, aloe vera not only helps the body's healing process, but also protects against infections that can occur in open wounds.

4. The B vitamins contained in aloe vera may help reduce the incidence, frequency, and severity of mood disorders and depression.

5. Providing a number of essential and nonessential amino acids, aloe vera can improve the body's muscle health.

6. When added to topical solutions, aloe vera's phytochemicals that allow for deeper penetration of the skin's layers may improve the effectiveness of topically applied creams, lotions, and medications.

7. With powerful phytochemicals that help reduce inflammation, aloe vera has been found to be an effective anti-inflammatory agent that can be ingested and applied topically, providing relief internally and externally.

8. With antiseptic benefits, aloe vera is able to help improve overall health by cleansing the blood and improving the functioning of all of the body's systems that receive nutrients via the bloodstream.

9. Aiding the body's absorption of essential vitamins and minerals, aloe vera can help reduce the risks of developing serious degenerative illnesses and diseases that affect the eyes, bones, skin, and organs.

10. Aloe vera is available in a number of forms that include powder, liquid, and gels.

Introduction

IN TODAY'S WORLD OF modern technology and medical advancements, it's hard to know if "natural" is really the best way to handle health. It seems like every day there's a new pharmaceutical creation or over-the-counter medication that can offer a "quick fix" to any trouble, symptom, illness, or disease. There are medications and "supplements" that not only promise to maintain your health but also to improve and enhance it.

Today we rely more and more on pharmaceutical companies for treatment options when it comes to our health. But, are processed and unnatural products the best way to handle health? Is relying on products, pills, and potions that may contain questionable ingredients—and that may or may not produce undesirable side effects—the way you want to handle your health?

For thousands of years, humankind relied on the earth to provide for life. Through natural healing treatments, handed down through generations and perfected with new advancements as they became available, humankind was able to live—happily, healthfully, and naturally. As time progressed, healers who relied on natural medicinal treatments for the care and curing of illnesses were phased out and considered less superior than their modern medicine contemporaries. Even today, those who recommend natural forms of medicine are referred to as administering "alternative medicine," as though it is less effective and less progressive than the methods utilized by pharmaceutical companies. This negative connotation could not be further from the truth.

With the advancements that have been made in research, technology, and communication, we can now see the value of natural healing methods more than ever. We now know the value of vitamin C in large doses in the fight against cancer, the power of B vitamins in the pursuit of happiness and mental health, the power of antioxidants in calming inflammation, and many more.

Knowing the importance of diet and the benefits that result from consuming the nutrients your body needs in order to function at its best, it is obvious that we need to revert back to natural sources—sources that improve the health of not just one organ or one symptom, but the whole body. We need to step away from the "one pill for every ill" mentality that seems to pervade our society.

Aloe vera has been used for hundreds of years for the treatment of many conditions, from skin ailments to digestive disorders. Its abundant vitamins and minerals and numerous phytochemicals combine to produce beneficial results in many areas of the body. Aloe vera is one of the few natural methods of healing that can actually improve quality of life, improve a specific system, or reduce the incidence of a specific health condition through either topical or consumed applications.

While you can never be completely and absolutely sure of the safety or side effects of pharmaceutical drugs, almost everyone can rely on the natural, safe, and profoundly effective benefits of aloe vera. Aloe vera transforms lives every day by healing wounds, optimizing system functioning, cleansing the blood, improving immunity, and prolonging life through the prevention of illness, disease, and degeneration. Aloe vera can play a major role in the prevention of health issues and the promotion of optimal health, effectively, safely, and naturally.

CHAPTER 1

A Long History of Use

Thousands of years ago, aloe vera held an important place in ancient cultures. Called the plant of immortality, the plant of harmony, and the royal plant, aloe vera was regarded as a gift from the gods to provide health, safety, security, and protection. Drawings on the walls of Egyptian temples depict the use of aloe to treat burns and other skin conditions. The army of Alexander the Great conquered a Somali island for the sole purpose of harvesting aloe vera to treat soldiers' wounds. The people of Mesopotamia believed aloe warded off evil spirits, and Native Americans called it the wand of heaven. Every part of the aloe plant was used to cure the sick, save the soul, and even help in the transition from life to death.

An Ancient Medicinal Plant

Aloe vera is a medicinal plant with a long history. It is depicted on the walls of ancient Egyptian temples, referenced in songs sung thousands of years ago, and frequently mentioned in the Bible. It was prized for its drought-resistant hardiness, its striking beauty, and especially its healing properties. It was used for a wide variety of medical treatments, and it was considered so important that aloe plants were placed in tombs for use in the afterlife. Even today it's one of the most popular natural remedies in use—found in skin treatments, digestive aids, and anti-inflammatory juices.

ESSENTIAL

It is believed that Cleopatra regularly used aloe vera as part of her beauty regimen. Her praise of aloe and its ability to maintain the beauty and youthfulness of her skin is in one of the earliest documented uses of the plant for skin care. Queen Nefertiti also used aloe vera—not only for beauty purposes, but also to support her digestive health.

It's remarkable that in a time when communication between continents was virtually nonexistent aloe vera was being used as an effective treatment for health issues in many different places. Ancient peoples could expect a short lifetime, often no more than 35–55 years. And without modern treatment, they often faced the possibility of death from something as simple as a cut or a burn. Aloe vera was a common option in a healer's limited medicine bag. It was effective in soothing skin irritation and burns, guarding against infections in cuts and gashes, and reducing inflammation of the throat and digestive tract. Used both externally and internally, aloe is believed to calm the respiratory and cardiovascular system, heal the skin, and treat constipation. And the gel has been used for centuries as one of the original beauty products.

Egypt

The use of aloe vera as a remedy can be traced back more than 6,000 years, to the ancient Egyptians. The plant is depicted in scrolls and on the walls of various places of worship. At this time, aloe was used externally to treat skin conditions, like cuts, burns, and rashes. It was also used as an internal treatment for digestive ailments including constipation, a common condition that in extreme forms could lead to fatal intestinal blockage. The juice of the plant, a powerful laxative, was prescribed to expel the demonic possessions believed to be causing the illnesses within.

FACT

The ancient Egyptians used aloe not only for its digestive benefits but also to fight against common but potentially deadly bacterial and viral infections, presumably extending their lifespans.

The antibacterial, antiviral, and antifungal properties of the aloe vera plant proved to be just as effective after death. The bodies of people whose skin had been treated with aloe vera seemed to decompose at a much slower rate than those who were not. This lead the Egyptians to believe that aloe vera assisted in the safe transport of the soul to the afterlife, leaving behind a perfectly preserved remembrance of the beloved. Because of this, Egyptians believed that the miracle plant was given to them by the gods, and it could protect them from not only afflictions of the body but also of the soul.

Ancient China and Japan

Aloe vera has been used in Asia since 400–300 B.C. Called *lu-hui* by the Chinese, aloe was initially used to heal rashes, skin irritations, burns, and lacerations. Healers ground up the leaves and boiled them to create a black gel that was applied to the skin. Aloe was used to treat wounds sustained in battle, to ward off infection, and to provide protection from spiritual harm.

Ancient Chinese writings of the Song Dynasty reveal that the Chinese began to experiment with the internal use of aloe around A.D. 700. It was considered an effective remedy for constipation and chronic indigestion, as well as respiratory and sinus conditions. In a time when illnesses and diseases were considered a punishment from the spiritual world, the healing properties of aloe warranted it a place as a valued natural remedy that could not only help restore health, but also protect against evil spirits and bad luck. Aloe, known as the plant of harmony, has been a widely accepted remedy for afflictions for centuries.

The use of aloe as a healing plant spread to Japan, where it was known as the royal plant. The first edition of the *Japanese Pharmacopoeia* (published in 1886) refers to the widespread use of aloe vera, calling aloe "the plant to make a doctor needless." Experimenting with its forms and applications, the Japanese produced treatment methods that utilized the juice from the aloe plant's fresh leaves. Japanese healers promoted the juice as a healing tonic—the most effective treatment for everything from gastric issues like constipation to skin abrasions and lacerations. Hundreds of years later, aloe was used to treat severe burns and wounds caused by radiation during World War II.

The Spread of Aloe to the World

How could one plant come to be so widely used, for almost every health condition imaginable by various cultures in countries on opposite sides of the earth? How could this one plant establish itself as a magical healer in cultures that had limited (if any) communication with one another in ancient times? Carried for miles, transported on ships, and traded in the economies of ancient civilizations, aloe vera spread like wildfire from one area of the world to the rest. Its powerful healing powers, various applications, and techniques for its use were conveyed by word of mouth and the written word.

A Widely Traveled Plant

The use of aloe vera in early medical practices spread from Egypt and Africa to Greece, India, Europe, and the Americas. Aloe's effectiveness in combating bacteria, viruses, and fungi made it a valuable medicine everywhere, since untreated infections could often result in death in a matter of days. As word spread, cultures around the world sought out aloe and began growing and harvesting their own. Because of its effectiveness in such a wide variety of treatment methods, aloe vera was packed on horseback, stored in the saddlebags of camels, and cultivated in pots on the decks of wide-traveling ships to be transported throughout the world by common travelers and famous conquerors alike.

ESSENTIAL

Many early cultures were nomadic, traveling across expansive, unfamiliar lands. With little room to carry anything other than the absolute essentials, it is surprising to learn that these people would include aloe vera plants among them. Carrying the plants with them as they traveled ensured that the aloe vera they used for numerous treatments would be readily available.

Writings, psalms, and spoken tales helped communicate the natural capabilities of aloe vera throughout the world.

The Aloe Industry

Today, aloe vera is growing in popularity, and its use has created one of the largest botanical industries around the globe. Just ten years ago, the industry for aloe vera tipped the scales of economic production by exceeding $125 million annually just for the purchase of the raw product, and people in the United States spent over $110 billion annually for products containing aloe. In today's modern world of production, aloe vera is used to create cosmetic, pharmaceutical, and food products. Included in the manufacturing of everything from skin creams, soaps, and sunblock to toilet paper, pills, and alcoholic beverages, aloe vera has evolved from a decorative plant to a multi-industry staple.

Early Documented Uses

The earliest written evidence of aloe vera being used as a medicine is found on a Sumerian clay tablet from 2200 B.C., which describes the aloe vera plant as having miraculous healing properties. The Ebers Papyrus, an ancient Egyptian medical document from 1550 B.C., is the first writing to include detailed descriptions of aloe vera, the numerous varieties, and its extensive medicinal value. While the information contained within the Ebers Papyrus is impressive in that the author was able to detail the plant's uses and applications, it surprises medical professionals to this day with its lengthy exploration of treatment methods. It includes twelve formulas combining aloe vera with other ingredients, designed specifically to treat unique internal and external disorders.

FACT

Alexander the Great (356–323 B.C.), on the advice of Aristotle, set out to conquer the island of Socotra, off the coast of Somalia, in order to control the cultivation of vast fields of aloe vera. The harvested aloe was sent to the battlefield for the treatment of soldiers' wounds and burns. Some people believe that Alexander's great military success was due in some part to the use of aloe, the miracle healer, to reduce losses in the aftermath of battles.

Dioscorides of Greece wrote in A.D. 70 about aloe vera's pharmacological effects, detailing its unique properties in depth. In the *Greek Herbal*, he chronicled his findings during years of traveling to research the medical and therapeutic healing properties of plants. Dioscorides determined that aloe vera was the most effective natural treatment for everything from topical applications for hair loss, genital ulcers, hemorrhoids, wounds and burns, to internal conditions ranging from gingivitis, tonsillitis, gastrointestinal discomfort, and parasitic invasions of the gut. Dioscorides wrote about aloe vera in many of his later books and promoted it as one of his favorite treatment methods.

In 1494, Christopher Columbus received a letter from his doctor, Diego Alvarez Chanca, while on his second voyage to the Americas that mentioned aloe vera and its remarkable spread to other lands. Dr. Chanca told Columbus, "A species of aloe we doctors are using is now growing in the Hispaniolas." Columbus is known to have carried ample amounts of aloe on each of his voyages. He was a major believer and promoter of aloe vera's benefits, sharing the plant with the people of the lands to which he traveled. According to Columbus, "Four vegetables are indispensable for the well-being of man: wheat, the grape, the olive, and aloe. The first nourishes him, the second raises his spirit, the third brings him harmony, and the fourth cures him."

In the Americas, aloe vera did not become popular within the medical community until well into the eighteenth century. Because the effectiveness of aloe vera declines while in transport, it did not become widely used until the growth and cultivation of American aloe was well established and the effectiveness of the plant in treatment methods was observed firsthand. In 1820, aloe vera was officially included in the most well-regarded medical document of its time, the *US Pharmacopoeia*, as a skin protectant and laxative. More than 100 years later, in 1930, aloe vera became well known in the Americas, with scientific studies backing the plant's effectiveness in treating radiation burns to the skin. By the mid-twentieth century, aloe was found in commercial products ranging from lotions and cosmetics to commonly prescribed treatments for chronic conditions.

Traditional Medicinal Uses

With 6,000 years of history, aloe vera has a long line of traditional uses that spans cultures and continents. While many cultures used aloe vera in similar ways, aloe vera's uses differed depending upon the type of aloe available, the climate, and the form used for the applications.

Egyptian

Ancient Egyptians used aloe vera to treat a number of issues, but the most common applications focused on gastric conditions, skin irritations and inflammations, and the preservation of the dead.

Chinese

Well-documented uses of aloe vera in Chinese medicine show that healers utilized the boiled and reduced black gel form of aloe vera to treat fungal diseases, sinus and respiratory issues, and skin conditions that resulted from radiation and burns.

India

In India, aloe vera was used in a variety of forms and showed to be an effective treatment for young and old. Colicky babies were remedied with aloe, as well as anyone suffering from constipation and gastric issues, parasitic infestations, and infections resulting from bacteria, fungi, viruses, and various microbes.

Mexico

Having embraced aloe vera far later than many other cultures, Mexico is one of the first countries to use aloe vera in creating effective treatment methods aiming to cure type 2 diabetes and minimize the symptoms associated with the disease.

Trinidad and Tobago

Scientists in Trinidad and Tobago were among the first to study the use of aloe vera in treating hypertension, having observed the well-known calming effect of aloe that is still utilized today in sleep aids.

The Americas

Able to withstand the dry and desert-like conditions of the land during certain seasons, aloe vera became a popular plant to the Native Americans. Referred to as the wand of the heavens, the Native Americans used aloe in a variety of treatments for skin conditions and gastric issues.

Modern Medicinal Uses

Today, aloe vera is used to treat conditions that affect the body both externally and internally. Aloe vera can provide relief for everything from scrapes and burns to major irritations and serious conditions. Research is now being conducted to study aloe's ability to help regenerate damaged skin cells, relieve symptoms of painful psoriasis, and even reduce the risk of skin cancer.

Ongoing Research

Memorial Sloan Kettering Cancer Center is currently studying aloe for potential effects on psoriasis and other skin issues, along with internal issues like constipation and diabetes.

There are studies going on today looking at aloe vera's effect on almost every condition that impacts the body's organs, systems, and even brain functioning. Aloe vera may hasten healing after periodontal treatments, according to the *Journal of Indian Society of Periodontology*, and it's believed to reduce blood sugar and total cholesterol levels while increasing "good cholesterol" levels (American College of Angiology). British studies show that aloe decreases irritation and enhances healing and repair of ulcers in the stomach and intestines. Aloe vera juice also helps decrease inflammation in irritable bowel syndrome, colitis, and other inflammatory disorders of the gut. Additionally, aloe vera can increase healthy bacteria in the intestines that aid digestion (*British Journal of General Practice*).

ESSENTIAL

Cats and dogs can also experience skin conditions as a result of nutritional deficiencies, underlying conditions, and exposure to environmental elements. Studies have shown that skin conditions in pets can be improved or even cured through the use of all-natural (and safe) aloe vera.

Aloe vera contains antibacterial, antiviral and antifungal properties that aid the immune system in cleansing the body of toxins and invading pathogens. Additionally, aloe vera helps balance the immune system to reduce the effects of seasonal allergies, rheumatoid arthritis, and other inflammatory immune disorders, according to the *Journal of Environmental Science and Health*.

Chronic Diseases

While aloe vera treatments for skin, gastric, and respiratory conditions are well documented in ancient history, researchers are currently exploring the possibility that aloe vera's potent naturally occurring properties may serve as part of an effective treatment method for serious diseases like cancer or AIDS. Possessing the powerful compounds that provide antibacterial, antiviral, antifungal, and antimicrobial effects, the aloe vera plant may be one of the few natural sources that can treat common conditions as well as possibly hold the key to unlocking the most evasive and difficult-to-treat health conditions this world has seen.

An All-Natural Daily Supplement

While these studies take time and there is a lot of scientific evidence and research needed before a stamp of approval can be placed on the implementation of an all-natural treatment such as this, for thousands of years the use of aloe vera has shown to be effective in treating a number of health issues.

More research is needed to support an FDA-approved supplement, a widely prescribed pharmaceutical, or even a generally accepted natural treatment alternative. But in the meantime, you can use this book to educate yourself on aloe's properties, uses, and supporting statistics and research to draw your own conclusions as to whether aloe vera can help you improve your quality of life. With 6,000 years of documented use, praise, and science behind it, aloe vera may just be the key to your health and vitality!

CHAPTER 2

Aloe Vera: The Healing Plant

While many people across the world have an aloe vera plant in or around their home, few know any information relating to the miracle plant's makeup, uses, applications, or benefits. With its natural form available year-round, regardless of your location on the globe, aloe vera can easily be grown, harvested, and applied. Requiring little attention and even less effort, your aloe plant can provide you with year-round benefits . . . all while providing you with a beautiful centerpiece that fits perfectly indoors or out!

Anatomy of the Aloe Plant

Most people know aloe as a plant that requires little to no attention or care, which is true of many of the aloe varieties. Because of the unique structure of the plant, aloe is able to withstand hot, cold, excessive or minimal water availability, and a wide variety of ground qualities that range from mineral-rich soil to soil-void dry rock formations. Because several parts of the aloe plant have distinct structures and uses, it is helpful to have an understanding of the parts of the plant and the products created from each.

Roots

In contrast to other plants whose root systems grow down deep into the soil, aloe roots spider into the ground and remain close to the top of its ground cover. This natural design of the plant allows the roots to better absorb any available moisture (in the forms of precipitation and condensation), store that water for later use, and become self-sustaining in times when little or no water is available. These string-like formations of thick roots are normally the circumference of an earthworm, and not only provide the main aloe plant with sustenance, but also produce offshoots of new growth. These new offshoots are not just extensions of the original plant, but are entirely new plants that can be removed and replanted individually.

FACT

While an aloe plant's root system may be condensed and remain relatively close to the surface of the soil, it is imperative that potted aloe plants are provided with adequate room for the plant's root system to grow. A pot that provides room for 3–5 times the original size of the root system should be sufficient for growth for up to 1–2 years.

Stem

Aloe is sometimes mistakenly referred to as a stemless plant, but the aloe does in fact have a stem that serves as its base. The aloe's stem grows larger and thicker with passing years, becoming more and more visible as the plant matures and grows in size. The stem is an important part of the aloe plant. It channels nutrients from the roots to the leaves, and it provides the leaves with a strong core from which they can grow securely. It is important that the stem is not compromised by extreme conditions in order to protect the life of the plant and the quality of its aloe.

FACT

Because the aloe plant grows actively between the months of April and October, your plant should be watered more regularly (about four times per month) and fertilized more consistently (about four times per month) in order to optimize the health of the plant.

Leaves

The leaves of the aloe plant grow in a variety of shapes, colors, and formations. Ranging in shades from dark to light green, aloe leaves are as different in appearance as the aloe plant is in number of species. Sometimes short and stubby, the leaves can also grow long and sword-like. Some varieties have obvious dark-colored or white spines on the sides of the leaves, while others have short, stubby, rounded leaves without spines. Appearing with speckles of color, delightful shades of blue or pink, and ranging in thickness from paper-thin to inches thick, aloe's design is most often specific to the type of environment from which the plant originates. It is also within the leaves that the aloin and pulp can be found.

Aloin

The yellow-colored sap that seeps from the leaves when cut is called aloin. Latex based, this potent element of the aloe leaf is actually considered by many to be an irritant to humans and possibly even toxic to pets. Many sources suggest handling leaves with care when aloin is seeping from the cut portions. Surprisingly, it is this product of aloe plants that is processed into the common laxatives used to restore or promote regularity.

Pulp

The actual pulp of the aloe plant is what most people picture when they think of aloe. When an aloe leaf is cut, the pulp is the clear substance resembling a gel. The meat of the leaf (simply the solidified form of the pulp) can be stripped away from the leaf, and the gel-like substance that surrounds the clear meat is what is referred to as the pulp. This portion of the aloe leaf is what is used to heal skin irritations and burns, and can be consumed for a wide variety of internal applications as well.

Stalk

A number of varieties of aloe have a stalk that grows out of the center. The stalk is a purple, brown, red, or white growth that can exceed 3' in height. Most often, this stalk will produce flowers in a variety of colors specific to the type of aloe from which it formed. This stalk's flowers can easily produce a number of quality seeds that can be used for further propagations of the plant.

Flowers

While beautiful, the red, orange, yellow, gold, and white flowers of the aloe plant have a very specific and important job: to create more aloe. The aloe plant's flowers are responsible for producing and spreading the seeds that produce new life. New aloe plants can also be produced manually by separating the flowery offshoots from the root system.

Aloe Plant Varieties

The aloe plant is a perennial succulent belonging to the lily family. Scientifically termed *Aloe barbadensis Miller*, the best-known variety of aloe is just one of the more than 400 species of aloe grown worldwide (with well over 100 interspecies crossbreeds). Among those many species of aloe, though, there is a specific group that has shown to be the most popular for decorative use as well as in the production of aloe for medicinal use and consumer consumption.

Among the most popular varieties of aloe are *Aloe vera L.*, *Aloe mutabilis*, *Aloe saponaria*, *Aloe brevifolia*, *Aloe ferox*, *Aloe descoingsii*, *Aloe spicata*, and *Aloe variegata*. The different varieties of aloe are as diverse as one could possibly imagine: some forms grow no taller than 6–10" and others grow in excess of 60'; some flower and others do not; and some are able to survive in the warmest climates with the heaviest rainfall measurements, while others are able to thrive in frigid temperatures or arid conditions. Following is a brief introduction to a few of the many aloe species to show you the differences in location, size, and production.

Aloe Vera L.

Aloe vera L. ("true aloe") produces a large plant with a short stem. This rosette perennial succulent has pale grayish-green leaves that resemble swords, which grow to about 80 cm in length. The larger varieties of the plant produce yellow tubular flowers. This variety is normally found in tropical areas, as it can't survive frosty conditions.

Aloe Ferox

This variety, also known as bitter aloe, produces green leaves with a blue hue that can reach heights of 2–3 meters. Its thick leaves are lined with reddish-brown teeth. The flowers that bloom from the plant's subspecies (*Aloe candelabrum*) in the winter months form a candelabra shape and are yellow, orange, or red in color. This aloe is best known for its medicinal qualities. Cultivated and harvested in South Africa, this aloe has a yellow sap beneath its skin that is referred to as Cape aloe and is used in most pharmaceutical applications as well as cosmetics.

Aloe Mutabilis

Aloe mutabilis, or krantz aloe, produces multiheaded succulent shrubs. The short stalks have large, lighter-colored teeth and produce beautiful yellow, orange, and red flowers during the winter months. The South African term *krantz* refers to the rocky areas of its origin. Surprisingly enough, this variety is the most commonly cultivated aloe and is the form that is found in most gardens with decorative appeal.

Aloe Saponaria

Known as haw aloe, this variety produces a centered main rosette that is surrounded by offshoots of smaller rosettes. The main rosette and its offshoots grow to a height and width of only 45 cm. Its lance-shaped succulent leaves are thick and green, with white speckles and dark brown teeth, and its center produces a beautiful purple stalk in the summer. Its tubular flowers are vibrant shades of yellow, orange, or red.

Aloe Brevifolia

Aloe brevifolia (blue aloe) is a striking plant. It produces a compact head of about 10 small rosettes that grow to only 50 cm. The leaves are a beautiful green with a pink hue, and have a thick line of white teeth along the leaves' sides. With vibrant orange and red flowers that grow in the fall and winter months, this variety of aloe can only be found in coastal areas that receive abundant rainfall and have rocky hillsides.

Aloe Spicata

This aloe, of the Baker subspecies, is best known for being the aloe from which the highest-quality medical-grade aloes are derived. This round, stubby plant has a short stem and grows to be an average of 1 meter high. It has leaves in the shape of wedges and unique white flowers that form the shape of bells as they hang downward.

Aloe Variegata

Aloe variegata (tiger aloe) only grows to a height of about 30 cm and has distinct rosettes that top one another as they grow, forming stacks of dark green rosettes and red flowers. Requiring little care, little water, and minimal sun exposure, this variety of aloe is the most common decorative aloe found in homes. Their height and slow growth make this aloe variety perfect for display on windowsills.

Growing Aloe

Throughout the world, aloe vera is cultivated, harvested, and utilized in a variety of climates. Able to thrive in the harshest of elements, the aloe vera plant can sustain itself in temperatures below freezing and up to temperatures in excess of 105°F.

Aside from extreme temperatures, aloe vera is also able to endure dry and wet conditions that would wipe out almost every other plant. Known to thrive in the tropics and subtropics, aloe vera has been able to survive in areas of the rainforest with excessive rainfall without the plant being damaged, so long as the root system of the plant is not destroyed. Not surprisingly, the plant is also able to survive in arid areas of the desert that receive minimal rainfall because of its ability to store water in its roots and leaves for later use. Most aloe is grown and farmed organically, which is possible because of the plant's natural ability to repel insects and fungi and withstand other challenges that commonly destroy crops.

The cultivation of aloe is a multibillion-dollar industry. Aloe crops are grown regionally in California, Texas, and Florida, and in large numbers throughout the world. While the common aloe houseplant requires little attention, growing aloe on a commercial level is very involved and includes a number of careful and precise measures and provisions. Growers must provide the optimal humidity, temperature, and soil for the growth of the plant from a seedling, while also ensuring that the water-packed plant receives adequate amounts of nutrients and hydration through soil propagation and irrigation.

ALERT

While the frigid temperatures that can kill other crops barely affect the aloe plant, you can safeguard your aloe from unnecessary exposure by paying particular attention to the months in which you water the plant's base. The months of April through September are fine for watering, but October through March watering should be minimized to just 1–2 times per month.

After the seedlings grow to a self-sustaining plant consisting of 2 or 3 nodes, they can be moved to the prepared field in which they will mature. The aloe plant quickly develops into rosettes of leaves that can vary in color. The small rosette formation develops from its stout base a number of larger leaf nodules that quickly turn into the aloe leaves with which you are most familiar. Set into acres of 5,000 plants or more, aloe thrives in the organized manufacturing setting, producing an average of 130,000 pounds of aloe per acre per year.

When cultivating the aloe vera's growths or "shoots" that can be self-sustaining to an area of soil, it is important to allow the cut growth to callus over for 2–5 days prior to planting. When the growth is ready for planting, simply place the growth atop the soil and mist with water weekly; overwatering at this stage will only cause rotting, not growth.

With so many varieties within its genus, it is surprising that the aloe plant has just two popular species that are used as the main source for production of the aloe-infused products used today. These include the aloe plants used to create the crude drug form of aloe, and the aloe plants that contain the gel or liquid that is used for consumption and in the treatment of internal and external issues.

Harvesting Aloe

The usable form of aloe vera moves from cultivation to harvest in just 18–24 months. The leaves are ready for harvest when the plant has flowered and there are enough large leaves that the common three-leaf removal (performed four times annually) will not disturb the growth or adversely affect the health of the plant. After the plant is suitable for harvesting, it is processed using either the whole-leaf method or the separation method, depending upon the projected use of the aloe harvested. Each method has its own benefits and drawbacks.

Whole-Leaf Method

The whole-leaf method refers to the processing of the entire aloe leaf in an effort to extract the juice. In this method, the commercial producers cut, mince, grind, and press the entire leaf of the aloe plant to create a pulp. The pulp then undergoes a filtration process using various sizes of filters or a charcoal-filter method. Following the filtering of the aloe, which often leaves behind numerous bits of the aloe leaf, the juice that is produced is processed using extreme cold or heat to destroy any impurities left behind.

As with most things, there are pros and cons to the whole-leaf method. The benefits of this method are that it tends to produce a high yield of aloe vera gel in a relatively short amount of time. The biggest downside to the whole-leaf method is its affect on the quality of the aloe vera gel produced. While the yields may be higher, the nutrient loss is huge. Another concern is that exposing the meat and gel of the aloe to the external leaf exudates causes contamination and degrades the bioavailable properties for which aloe is sought. Additionally, the filtering of the aloe consistently leaves bits of the aloe leaf behind, and the use of extreme temperatures actually kills a number of beneficial enzymes and micronutrients, leaving the aloe produced far inferior to aloes processed using the separation method.

Separation Method

Also known as the filleting method (as in "filleting a fish"), the separation method has been used for thousands of years and is still the favored method of aloe production today. In this method, the aloe is harvested and immediately brought to a station in which the separation takes place. The separation is done by machine or by hand. A knife or sharp tool is run along the underside of the leaf's exterior on each side, carefully revealing the intact meat and gel of the aloe. The gel (or sap) is allowed to drip from the leaf's underside and the exterior of the meat into a collection drum. Once the gel is collected, it is prepared for storage and distribution for use in a number of applications.

As with the whole-leaf method, there are benefits and drawbacks to the separation method. In terms of the amount of gel produced and the time required to process the leaves manually, the difference is dramatic, with the whole-leaf method producing far more product in far less time. Another drawback to the separation method involves the machines used to perform the separation. Because the machines compress and cut the leaves on a set scale (regardless of the length or thickness of the meat), the production often results in loss of gel, loss of meat, and possible interaction of the gel with the exudates of the leaf.

In terms of the benefits of the separation method, the aloe vera gel that is produced is of the highest quality, with care taken throughout the process to preserve the nutrients. Performed in less than 48 hours, the entire process of the manual separation method is designed to keep the nutrients intact and retain the plants bioavailability. This process does not utilize heating or cooling, so the aloe vera is not exposed to damaging conditions. The meat and gel are kept separate from the leaves and are not exposed to the leaf's exudates at any point, further minimizing the possibility of contamination.

With the application of aloe vera, internally or externally, the consumer is normally in search of a nutrient-dense aloe vera with optimal bioavailable enzymes and naturally occurring phytochemicals. By opting for an aloe vera product that is certified as being produced using the separation method by hand and without heat, you can ensure that your aloe vera will meet your expectations and provide you with the nutrients you would find in the aloe if you harvested it yourself.

CHAPTER 3

The Benefits of Aloe Vera

If you find yourself wondering what exactly is in the aloe plant that can provide such powerful benefits for such a wide range of illnesses and ailments, you're not alone. Scientists and researchers have spent decades looking into the exact science behind the aloe plant's effectiveness and have determined that the inconspicuous aloe plant contains a surprising number of vitamins, minerals, and specialized phytochemicals that come together synergistically to improve the body's health on even the seemingly most insignificant cellular level. With every one of these naturally occurring elements helping to improve the health and recovery of the body, aloe's vital nutrients should get the recognition each deserves.

Vitamins

Vitamins play a major role in every aspect of how your body and brain function—ranging from nerve impulses to muscle contractions to clarity of mind to lasting energy, and even the quality of your sleep. In fact, the Food and Drug Administration (FDA) and the United States Department of Agriculture (USDA) have identified the following thirteen specific vitamins as imperative for optimal health:

- Vitamin A (carotenoids)
- Vitamin B_1 (thiamine)
- Vitamin B_2 (riboflavin)
- Vitamin B_3 (niacin)
- Vitamin B_5 (pantothenic acid)
- Vitamin B_6 (pyridoxine)
- Vitamin B_7 (biotin)
- Vitamin B_9 (folic acid)
- Vitamin B_{12} (cobalamin)
- Vitamin C
- Vitamin D
- Vitamin E
- Vitamin K

Many of these vitamins can be found in aloe vera. Aloe contains vitamin B_{12}, folic acid, choline, and vitamins A, C, and E.

ALERT

For every vitamin's benefit, there is an equally consequential dysfunction that can result from a lack of it. For example, vitamin B is well known to help with metabolic functioning and energy production and maintenance. With regular consumption of nutritious foods that contain vitamin B, people feel the benefits in their energy levels and metabolism; on the contrary, a deficiency of vitamin B results in a slower or irregular metabolism and a negative fluctuation in energy levels.

But before you learn how each vitamin will affect your body, it's important for you to know that there are two classifications of vitamins: water-soluble and fat-soluble.

Water-soluble vitamins—which include all the B vitamins and vitamin C—are easily dissolved in water and in your bloodstream. Because their excesses are flushed out on a regular basis in your urine, you need a consistent renewal of these vitamins daily.

Fat-soluble vitamins—which include vitamins A, D, E, and K—are first absorbed by your body's fat stores before entering the bloodstream to perform their functions. Each of these vitamins serves a different purpose in your body's functioning, so it is of the utmost importance that you get a certain amount of each on a regular basis. However, because the excesses of these vitamins are stored in the liver, it is important not to exceed the recommended amount.

The suggested daily values of some of the vitamins discussed in this chapter can vary depending on the specific needs of each individual. For example, pregnant women have very different needs than elderly males. They may fluctuate as well depending upon certain individual conditions, such as weight, lifestyle, and age. However, the need for them remains constant for every body and every life.

Vitamin A (Carotenoids)

Fat-soluble vitamins that start out as carotenoids (the orange pigments of plants) are transformed into vitamin A when your body needs it. Important to the immune system and to the development of red blood cells, vitamin A is an essential element, especially for pregnant women (it helps in the healthy development of a fetus). Vitamin A also aids in the synthesis of your body's proteins and helps your eyes by preventing premature aging, free radical damage, and diseases specific to the eyes. In addition to aloe vera, this vitamin can be found in a wide variety of deep orange, yellow, green, and red fruit and vegetables, as well as in certain milks and milk products such as almond milk, cow's milk, and yogurt.

Vitamin B$_9$ (Folic Acid)

Vitamin B$_9$ (also known as folic acid or folate) is a water-soluble vitamin that helps optimize blood functions like production and circulation. It is an important vitamin that you need to include in your daily diet. This vitamin is especially important for people suffering from iron deficiencies and women who are nursing, pregnant, or may become pregnant because it works to improve the absorption of iron and to ensure the proper development of a growing fetus. Some great sources of vitamin B$_9$ include:

- Asparagus
- Beans
- Beets
- Cauliflower
- Citrus fruit
- Lettuce
- Spinach
- Whole grains

Vitamin B$_{12}$ (Cobalamin)

Vitamin B$_{12}$ (also known as cobalamin) is a water-soluble vitamin that is best known for its promotion of energy and metabolic maintenance. In addition to optimizing the body's metabolic processes, vitamin B$_{12}$ is also absolutely necessary in red blood cell production and in the formation and maintenance of healthy nerve cells. Many people opt for a B$_{12}$ supplement (which is most often recommended in a sublingual liquid form or a shot), but this vitamin can easily be absorbed through natural sources.

ESSENTIAL

While many plants provide the full spectrum of essential vitamins, very few provide the much-needed vitamin B$_{12}$, cobalamin. Aloe vera is one of the few that not only provides a number of beneficial B vitamins, but also contributes B$_{12}$! The number of plants that provide the full range of vitamins is small. Aloe vera's ability to provide all the essentials (including every single B vitamin) makes it stand out from the crowd.

Vitamin C

A water-soluble vitamin that is highly regarded as a protector of the immune system, vitamin C works as a multitasking agent for your body's overall health. Aside from boosting the body's defenses by acting as a strong antioxidant (a disease-fighting property found in plants, fruit, and vegetables) that fights damaging free radicals, vitamin C plays a crucial part in the absorption of iron, the regeneration of vitamin E, and the development and regeneration of the body's collagen. While many people reach for citrus sources to replenish their vitamin C stores, it can also be obtained from a wide array of other natural foods, including:

- Asparagus
- Bell peppers
- Broccoli
- Cauliflower
- Citrus fruit
- Green leafy vegetables
- Kiwifruit
- Mangoes
- Papayas
- Peas
- Potatoes
- Strawberries

Vitamin E

Vitamin E is a fat-soluble vitamin that is highly regarded as a strong antioxidant capable of correcting the damage done by free radicals, which are damaging chemicals that can alter the growth of healthy cells. In addition to the way it works to correct the damage to the body's cells, vitamin E plays an important role in the communication between the body's cells by keeping fluid levels and cell environments clear and healthy. All these disease-fighting abilities help your body maintain healthy blood quality, bone structure, and muscle tissue. Some great sources of vitamin E include:

- Apples
- Avocados
- Carrots
- Green leafy vegetables
- Nuts
- Tomatoes
- Vegetable oils
- Whole grains

Minerals

Minerals are another major support network that betters the body's functioning. Minerals assist in everything from developing and strengthening teeth and bones to optimizing the quality and volume of our blood; they are a necessary nutrient that we have to get from outside sources. Aside from carrying out their own individual tasks, most minerals actually support the roles of other minerals and promote health through a symbiotic relationship that improves the quality of each. For example, calcium is absolutely necessary for strong teeth and bones, and fluorine acts as a support system for calcium's hard work by providing the teeth with added protection against tooth decay. Hand in hand, each of the following ten minerals recognized by the Food and Drug Administration (FDA) and the United States Department of Agriculture (USDA) as being needed on a daily basis plays an important role in ensuring that your body runs at its best each and every day:

- Calcium
- Copper
- Iron
- Magnesium
- Manganese
- Phosphorous
- Potassium
- Selenium
- Sodium
- Zinc

While there are many supplements available that can provide synthetic forms of many minerals, getting those minerals from natural food sources is always the better (and safer) alternative. Aloe vera contains several of these vital minerals, including calcium, zinc, selenium, magnesium, chromium, copper, manganese, potassium, and sodium.

Calcium

This important mineral is most often associated with (a) healthy teeth and bones, and (b) dairy products. This correlation isn't off base, but the functions and sources of calcium aren't that limited. Calcium also promotes proper hormone release and regulation. It also improves the quality of nerve impulses in all the body's systems, helping the brain and body communicate with each other efficiently. Without them functioning at their best, your reflexes, muscle contractions, and thought processes would all suffer. Adequate calcium intake is essential for the overall health of your body. Some great sources of calcium include:

- Almonds
- Beans/lentils
- Broccoli
- Dairy products
- Green leafy vegetables
- Rhubarb
- Tofu
- Turnips

FACT

The body needs adequate amounts of calcium on a regular basis in order to maintain proper functioning. If there is not enough of a supply consumed through foods and liquids, your body taps into the calcium stores of the bones. If this continues for years, the bones weaken, and they can become susceptible to breakage, a disease known as osteoporosis.

Copper

Copper's relationship with its fellow mineral iron is so interdependent that the symptoms of copper deficiency are actually the same as iron deficiency (anemia). This mineral is of the utmost importance to the health of the blood and all its functions; without copper, red blood cell production and cell quality would be severely impaired. Copper also plays a major role in absorbing oxygen and supplying it to the bloodstream. The ever-important blood-supporting iron consumed in foods would not be adequately absorbed, stored, or metabolized by the body without the necessary amounts of copper available. In addition to all the support copper gives to our blood functions, it also acts as a strong antioxidant that can fight off free radical damage in healthy cells. Some great sources of copper include:

- Almonds
- Barley
- Cashews
- Garbanzo beans
- Lentils
- Mushrooms
- Navy beans
- Peanut butter
- Soybeans
- Tempeh
- Whole grains

ESSENTIAL

Like many other minerals, iron is greatly impacted by the presence or absence of other minerals and can influence the effectiveness of other minerals in the body. For optimal iron absorption, adequate copper levels need to be maintained. Vitamin C ingested at the same time improves the absorption of iron, while calcium ingested at the same time impairs the absorption of iron. In addition, when iron and zinc are consumed in the same meal, iron impairs the effectiveness of zinc.

Magnesium

Magnesium plays an important part in almost every body function, from insulin production and utilization to the generation of healthy cells, and from bone strength to proper blood clotting. It even affects the quality of the processing of B vitamins. Like so many other minerals, magnesium has a huge impact on the absorption of other minerals; by ensuring that your body has adequate levels of magnesium, you can ensure the quality absorption of potassium and calcium as well. Athletes and those who strive to gain better control of their body composition can also greatly benefit from increased attention to their intake of this essential mineral because, among other important tasks, magnesium makes the body's metabolism of carbohydrates and fats its main priority. In addition, this mineral supports the body's use and regeneration of DNA and RNA. Some great sources of magnesium include:

- Almonds
- Apples
- Apricots
- Bananas
- Black beans
- Cashews
- Green leafy vegetables
- Lima beans
- Molasses
- Navy beans
- Peanuts

Manganese

Although the full extent of manganese's effects on the body is still not as fully understood as some of the other minerals, its role in optimizing metabolic functions is an important one. By consuming adequate amounts of manganese, you ensure that the metabolic processes of absorbing, processing, storing, and utilizing all the macronutrients (including carbohydrates, proteins, fats, and cholesterols) is top-notch. This not only helps the body function at its best, but it also makes for more regular blood sugar levels, which can help everything from energy levels to brain functioning. While most people know little about manganese, its sources, and its benefits, it is important to note that this is a very important mineral that is a must in your diet. Some great sources of manganese include:

- Almonds
- Beans/lentils
- Cloves
- Oats
- Peanuts
- Pecans
- Pineapples
- Raspberries
- Spinach
- Sweet potatoes
- Tempeh

ALERT

The adequate intake of other minerals—including iron and calcium—is equally important as magnesium, but it's necessary to note that consuming supplements of these minerals together can reduce the effectiveness of the magnesium. Consequently, you should try to take your supplements of other minerals at different times of the day.

Potassium

Potassium's main priority is to maintain proper fluid balance within your body by keeping the fluid balance within all cells of the body at optimal levels. Adequate hydration is vital to survival, and without adequate levels of potassium to safeguard the body's hydration and cell functioning, all your body's systems would be severely impaired. The symptoms of inadequate potassium levels can range from a slight tingling in the hands and feet to muscle weakness to even severe vomiting and diarrhea. Some great sources of potassium include:

- Artichokes
- Bananas
- Green leafy vegetables
- Prunes
- Raisins
- Spinach
- Squash
- Tomatoes
- Yams and sweet potatoes

Selenium

Selenium works to maintain healthy cells by protecting them from free radical damage. When free radicals interact with healthy cells, transformations take place that cause the originally healthy cells to mutate into unhealthy cells; with too many unhealthy cells in the body, certain illnesses, such as cancers, can result. While selenium also aids in enzymatic activities throughout the body, its main role is to serve as an antioxidant that works hand in hand with vitamin E to protect your body's sensitive cells from harmful changes that could possibly turn normal cells into cancerous ones. Some great sources of selenium include:

- Milk
- Mushrooms
- Walnuts
- Whole grains
- Yogurt

Sodium

Sodium is heavily involved with maintaining proper fluid levels in the body, and it also regulates your body's blood volume and blood pressure. In addition, adequate levels of sodium ensure optimal absorption and use of the essential amino acids, other important minerals, and, of course, water! The good news is that by consuming adequate amounts of sodium through fruit, vegetables, nuts, and whole grains, you can ensure that your body is supplied with the right amounts and of the natural variety. But don't overdo it; many people suffer from sodium sensitivity, which can show itself with the uncomfortable symptoms of water retention and swelling in the hands, feet, and lower legs. Some great sources of sodium include:

- Fruit
- Nuts
- Vegetables
- Whole grains

Zinc

While zinc offers major benefits in bettering the functioning of almost all the body's systems, you may be surprised to hear that this mineral has to be present in order for all chemical reactions to take place; that means enzyme reactions, cell functioning, and everything from digestion to thought processes require zinc for optimal results. Getting adequate amounts of zinc can ensure that your body's processes function as intended. Some great sources of zinc include:

- Almonds
- Beans
- Cashews
- Garbanzo beans
- Mushrooms
- Peas
- Yogurt

FACT

Like many other vitamins and minerals whose effectiveness is affected by the supplementation or high intake of other minerals, zinc's potency is undermined by taking increased amounts of (or combining it with) folic acid, calcium, and iron.

Amino Acids

Appropriately referred to as the building blocks of the body, amino acids play an intricate role in processing a number of important elements. From the breakdown and utilization of carbohydrates, proteins, and fats, to fighting off illnesses and preventing dangerous changes from occurring within the body, amino acids are required in every bodily function. Amino acids are classified as either essential or nonessential depending upon whether the body is able to produce the amino acid on its own or is only able to acquire the amino acid from food. An essential amino acid is one that is absolutely necessary to the vital processes of the body but cannot be synthesized by the body; because the body is unable to produce these amino acids, it is essential that they be consumed in the diet. The nonessential amino acids are those that are produced by the body and do not need to be sought out in dietary forms. The most common sources of the essential amino acids are meat, eggs, dairy products, beans, and some whole-grain foods such as quinoa. Aloe vera is rich in amino acids and contains lysine, methionine, leucine, threonine, valine, tryptophan, isoleucine, and phenylalanine.

ESSENTIAL

The same amino acids utilized by the muscles to promote physical activity and maintain proper structure of the body do double duty by starring in the production of healthy hair. Without sufficient amounts of amino acids, both essential and nonessential, your hair can appear dull and lackluster and be prone to frizz and breakage.

Essential Amino Acids

- **Isoleucine:** a branched-chain amino acid (BCAA) used for energy by muscle tissue; plays an important part in the formation of hemoglobin
- **Leucine:** a branched-chain amino acid (BCAA) used as a source of energy, promoting the repair of skin and bone, and reducing muscle protein breakdown

- **Lysine:** an antiviral that combines with vitamin C to form L-carnitine, enabling muscles to effectively use oxygen and delay fatigue; aids in the formation of collagen and cartilage
- **Methionine:** reduces blood cholesterols, purges toxic waste from the liver, and assists in regeneration of organ tissue
- **Phenylalanine:** improves memory, learning processes, and mood and alertness; aids in collagen production and suppresses appetite; used to treat depression
- **Threonine:** prevents lipid buildup in the liver; essential in collagen production
- **Valine:** a branched-chain amino acid (BCAA) that is not processed by the liver; assists the brain in the uptake of neurotransmitters

Nonessential Amino Acids

Aloe vera also contains twelve nonessential amino acids, including alanine, arginine, asparagine, aspartic acid, cysteine, glutamic acid, glutamine, glycine, histidine, proline, serine, and tyrosine.

- **Alanine:** a major component of connective tissue; improves immunity, and helps processes that allow muscles and tissues retain energy from amino acids
- **Arginine:** balances the levels of insulin, glucagon, and hormones; improves collagen formation; acts as a neurotransmitter in the brain; aids in sufficient production of sperm
- **Aspartic acid:** helps convert carbohydrates to muscle energy, builds immunity by producing antibodies, and helps reduce ammonia levels and lactic acid levels after exercise
- **Cysteine:** detoxifies chemicals, stimulates white blood cell activity, and helps prevent damage sustained from alcohol and tobacco use
- **Glutamic acid:** a potential energy source that is important to the brain's metabolism and the metabolism of amino acids
- **Glutamine:** the most prominent amino acid, it improves immune system functioning and kidney function; an essential source of energy that promotes brain activity, assisting in memory and focus

- **Glycine:** aids in production of companion amino acids, produces glucagon, inhibits sugar cravings, and helps treat aggression and depression by producing a calming effect
- **Histidine:** absorbs UV light in the skin, plays a crucial part in production of red and white blood cells, and acts to combat inflammation
- **Proline:** aids in the formation of connective tissue; a major component in collagen, used as energy for muscles
- **Serine:** essential in energy production; improves memory and nervous system functioning, and improves immunity through antibody production
- **Tyrosine:** acts as a precursor for neurotransmitters (dopamine, epinephrine, and norepinephrine), improves hormone production and thyroid regulation, and improves mood; essential for formation of pigmentation (skin and hair color)

Enzymes

When any chemical reaction takes place in the body, an enzyme is involved. In order for the body's systems to communicate, for changes to take place, or for any type of imaginable activity (even thought processes), an enzyme is required. Regulating the body's immune system, hormone production, and even mood and stress levels, the enzymes that are required for every process in the body are acquired through the diet. With a poor diet that consists of heavily processed foods and lacking in quality nutrients from whole foods such as fruit, vegetables, and whole grains, the intake of the essential enzymes is minimal and results in insufficient enzymatic activity. Without the enzymes needed for all the body's systems to function properly, one's overall health can be adversely affected. You can obtain all the necessary enzymes from clean sources of food, including aloe, and maintain quality health naturally. The following ten enzymes are bountiful in minimally processed forms of aloe, such as cold-pressed liquids and gels, and can assist the body in a multitude of processes that improve overall health:

- **Alkaline phosphatase:** achieves an alkaline environment by removing phosphates from nucleotides, proteins, and alkaloids
- **Amylase:** breaks down sugars and starches
- **Bradykinin:** stimulates the immune system; provides anti-inflammatory and analgesic properties
- **Carboxypeptidase:** involved in blood clotting, wound healing, hormone production, and digestion, as well as the maturation of proteins
- **Catalase:** prevents excessive water accumulation in the body
- **Cellulase:** aids in the digestion of cellulose (fiber)
- **Creatine phosphokinase:** aids in the metabolic processes of the body
- **Lipase:** aids in the digestion of fats
- **Oxidase:** improves the utilization of oxygen
- **Protease (or peptidase):** assists in the digestion and utilization of protein

Anthraquinones

The bitter taste and yellowish coloring of aloe vera drinks and gels is provided by the rich anthraquinones of the aloe leaf. Responsible for improving the antimicrobial, antiviral, and antioxidant benefits of aloe, anthraquinones are found in high quantities in the aloe plant. These organic compounds not only help the body fend off inflammation and infections, but also prevent free radical damage to the cells. Anthraquinones seek and destroy free radicals, preventing their cancerous changes in cells that can lead to serious cancers throughout the body. With aloin, barbaloin, and aloe emodin being the three most potent of the anthraquinones, there are an impressive ten anthraquinones found in aloe that contribute powerful health-promoting benefits. Combining to create an effective all-inclusive prevention against health-deteriorating illnesses, these ten anthraquinones provide antiviral, antimicrobial, antibacterial, anti-inflammatory, and anti-oxidant properties:

- Aloe emodin
- Aloetic acid
- Aloin
- Anthracene
- Barbaloin

- Chrysophanic acid
- Emodin
- Ester of cinnamic acid
- Ethereal oil
- Resistanol

Phytochemicals Worth Mentioning

Phytochemicals are the naturally occurring chemicals found specifically in plants. In addition to the plentiful vitamins, minerals, amino acids, enzymes, and anthraquinones found in aloe, there are a number of additional phyto-chemicals provided by the aloe plant that are worth mentioning. Lignin, saponin, salicylic acid, saccharide, and sterol provide a variety of benefits that range from improving the effectiveness of aloe to cleansing the blood and improving immunity.

Lignins

Found in the cells of plants, lignins provide the structural component that allows a plant to stand upright. In aloe products, it is this component that aids in the absorption of aloe by the skin. Aloe and all its properties not only benefit the body's surface but also permeate to the circulatory system and flow throughout the body.

Saponins

These compounds are often referred to as soapy compounds because of their ability to cleanse the blood of harmful elements. With antimicro-bial, antiviral, antibacterial, and antifungal properties, saponins are the anti-septic compounds of aloe that help protect and promote one's health while improving immune system functioning.

Salicylic Acid

This compound delivers aspirin-like effects by reducing inflammation, inhibiting pain receptors, fighting microbes and bacteria, and even reducing fevers.

Saccharides

With a number of naturally occurring monosaccharides and polysaccharides, the aloe plant provides two especially powerful elements that act to build immunity and fight disease. Acemannan and alprogen are immunostimulants that also act as anticarcinogenic and anti-inflammatory agents.

Sterols

Plant sterols act to minimize cholesterol by binding with cholesterol receptors in the blood and inhibiting those receptors from absorbing cholesterol. With impressive documented studies that show the effect of plant sterols on cholesterol levels can be as high as a 9–14 percent reduction in LDL cholesterol and a 10 percent reduction in overall cholesterol, sterols are being considered a possible breakthrough in the reduction of heart disease. In addition to cardiovascular benefits, the sterols of aloe vera act as powerful anti-inflammatory agents that can help alleviate pain, inhibit swelling, and reduce the incidence of harmful health changes that can result from chronic inflammation.

Aloe Vera and Immunity

Without a healthy immune system, it doesn't matter what you do for the promotion of health among your body's systems, because one illness that isn't defended against can quickly ravage the body, affecting every system. The immune system is the first line of defense and the biggest support system for the protection and proper functioning of the body. Providing protection against the most common of colds to the most severe ailments that can wreak havoc on your body, your immunity is, arguably, the most important aspect of health.

When a microbe, bacteria, virus, or fungus is introduced to your body, your immune system moves into action, recruiting the white blood cells to attack the foreign invader. This reaction then calls the cardiovascular system into play, with the blood carrying the germs and any damaged cells to the digestive system to be purged from the body.

Two of the most common symptoms that result from the contraction of a harmful irritant like germs, bacteria, and viruses are diarrhea and vomiting, which are the body's natural processes of purging the harmful illness-causing irritants. Following the fight against the illness, the immune system moves into repair mode, restoring lost nutrients, electrolytes, and hydration to the body's cells and utilizing antioxidant support to maintain the health of cells throughout the body.

The immune system's functioning is supported greatly by the introduction of aloe vera. Whether you choose to treat a cut with aloe vera or ingest 2 ounces of the liquid version daily, aloe vera can help improve your immune system's functioning through protection and prevention. With powerful nutrients and phytochemicals that help fight germs, prevent infection, fight inflammation, aid in repair processes, and help in restoring the normal functioning of cells, organs, and systems, aloe vera can be a helpful aid in preventing illness and disease, ensuring that the quality of your life is protected.

Infection Protection

Infections can occur anywhere. Any cell, tissue, organ, or system can fall victim to an illness or disease that starts with an unnoticeable infectious microbe. While taking certain precautions like hand washing and even maintaining oral health can help safeguard against infections, the body should receive support from antibacterial, antiviral, antimicrobial, and antioxidant-rich agents like those found in aloe vera.

Through its provision of powerful phytochemicals that combine to fight these illness creators, aloe vera can help protect the body against infection at every line of defense. Topically, aloe vera can be applied to skin to prevent infectious agents from being able to enter through cuts, scrapes, and burns, while also preventing them from being able to survive or thrive on the skin's surface.

Ingested Protection

When ingested, aloe vera is able to provide protection against infection by supporting the cardiovascular, digestive, lymphatic, and immune systems with those same powerful phytochemicals that fight against microbes, bacteria, and viruses. Once these infectious agents are able to travel past the first line of defense and infiltrate the body, the spread of infection is delivered throughout the body by way of the bloodstream, and then through multiple systems' communication. By ingesting aloe vera, the properties responsible for providing protection against infectious agents are delivered directly to the body's systems, organs, and cells within a matter of moments.

Internal Illness Prevention

With millions of cellular changes occurring throughout the brain and body every second, it's no wonder that illness and disease can take over a cell and then quickly spread throughout the body. Harmful cellular changes are caused by carcinogens, which cause cell dysfunction. The carcinogens change cells from healthy to unhealthy and then recruit surrounding cells to do the same. The key is to protect these cells from the carcinogens and prevent carcinogenic changes.

Through powerful antioxidants, aloe vera is able to support the protection of your cells. Specialized phytochemicals in aloe vera act as antiseptic agents, cleansing the blood of harmful infectious agents. Aloe vera is not only able to help in the fight against free radicals and carcinogens, but it is also able to provide support to the cardiovascular system so that it can purge the destroyed disease-causing agents and the damaged cells from the body.

CHAPTER 4

Skin Soothing

Since the beginning of humankind, skin ailments have been an issue that can not only be uncomfortable, but can also lead to illnesses, disease, and even in severe cases, death. Whether you experience a minor cut or burn, or develop a festering wound that is plagued with infection, aloe can be a surprisingly effective treatment method. Providing anti-inflammatory, antimicrobial, and immunity-boosting properties, aloe can be used topically and internally to safeguard your cut, burn, or irritation while improving and accelerating the healing of your wound. Current research and thousands of years of documented successful applications show that aloe is one of the most effective treatment methods in ailments of the skin.

The Skin

With a total surface area of about 20 square feet, your skin is the largest organ of your body. Designed to protect your body in a number of ways, the skin not only acts as a containment for all the blood, fluid, bones, and organs in your body, but it also aids in the protection of your body's systems against disease and the elements. In addition to helping regulate the body's temperature and provide the most sensitive of senses (touch), the skin helps provide information to your brain about the outside world. The skin does an efficient job of performing a multitude of tasks designed to keep the body safe, from acting as a barrier to providing communication between the environment and the brain. Skin is made up of multiple layers, with extra layers of skin on the soles of the feet and palms of the hands. The three main skin layers—the epidermis, the dermis, and the hypodermis—each provide the body with a different extent of health protection with subsequent components that promote health or protect against environmental factors.

Epidermis

The epidermis is the outermost layer of skin. This layer of skin provides the body with waterproof protection strong enough to create a barrier against liquids, solids, and particles in the environment. The epidermis contains pores that allow the absorption of trace elements from the environment. It is the layer of skin that is subject to the most exposure and sustains the most damage. This layer of skin contains the melanocytes that produce the pigment (melanin) that provides the body with skin color. The epidermis is also the portion of the skin that is most vulnerable to sun damage and cancerous changes that may result.

ESSENTIAL

By ingesting aloe vera on a regular basis, it is possible to not only improve the functioning of the entire body, but also experience the beauty benefits of healthy skin. With daily aloe vera use, anyone can easily improve skin conditions and enjoy the benefits of maximized skin health.

There are three types of specialized cells in the epidermis: keratino-cytes, melanocytes, and Langerhans cells. The keratinocytes help in the synthesis of specialized proteins in the epidermal layer of the skin called ker-atin; this protein is the strongest of all proteins in the skin and acts to form the rigidity and strength of the skin. The melanocytes produce the melanin that creates the skin's tone and color. The Langerhans cells act as strength-ening protection against foreign substances, helping to promote the skin's ability to remain "waterproof."

Including the two layers of skin that cover the soles of the feet and the palms of the hands (stratum corneum and stratum lucidum), the epidermis is composed of five layers of skin:

- Stratum corneum
- Stratum lucidum
- Stratum granulosum
- Stratum spinosum
- Stratum germinativum

Dermis

The layer of skin found directly beneath the epidermis is called the dermis and consists of two parts: the dermal papillary layer and the dermal reticular layer. This layer of skin is where connective tissue, hair follicles, and sweat glands are located. When you sense pain, temperature, or other sensations, it is due to the nerves located in your dermis. Also responsible for the formation of wrinkles, the dermis is where the specialized proteins, collagen and elastin, are found in high concentration.

Collagen is the most abundant protein in the body, making up a stagger-ing 75 percent of the skin. Synthesized by fibroblasts within the dermis, col-lagen and elastin are the source of support and elasticity in the skin. With age and environmental and lifestyle factors diminishing the body's ability to produce collagen and elastin, the skin shows signs of age in the form of wrinkles (resulting from insufficient collagen) and sagging (from insufficient elastin).

Due to aloe's unique ability to improve the body's production of the fibroblasts responsible for generating the collagen and elastin of the skin, aloe is not only able to effectively treat ailments and abrasions, but can also improve the skin's appearance by increasing the production of these two essential proteins.

Hypodermis

The hypodermis is the deepest subcutaneous skin layer that is made of fat and connective tissue. Responsible for maintaining the body's ideal temperature and protecting the body's internal organs from outside interference, the hypodermis is where the fatty cells, known as adipocytes, can be found. The fat storage that is within the hypodermis is absolutely essential in the body's thermoregulatory processes, energy production, and even in protecting the body from external injuries that could pose harm to the internal organs. An interesting fact about the hypodermis is that it tends to collect around specialized areas depending upon sex, with men showing excess hypodermis around their abdomen and women around their waist, thighs, and buttocks.

Scrapes, Cuts, and Bruises

The skin is the protective sheath that not only encapsulates your body's internal elements like blood, bones, veins, and organs, but it is also designed to protect your body and all its systems from foreign invaders like germs, bacteria, viruses, and so on. A simple bike ride or dinner preparation can easily result in a scraped knee or cut finger. With an increasing awareness about the infections that can occur as a result of lacerations of the skin (scrapes count as lacerations because the skin is broken, exposing the body to environmental elements), there is a growing interest in the most effective treatment methods for skin injuries that can help protect against not only common infections caused by germs, bacteria, and viruses, but also severe infections like staph. Luckily, aloe vera provides vitamins, minerals, and phytochemicals that act synergistically to improve the body's natural healing and speed healing time, and also protect against infections that can quickly turn a slight cut or scrape into something much more serious.

FACT

Using aloe vera to treat a skin irritation occurring from exposure to naturally irritating or poisonous plants such as poison ivy has proved to be beneficial in most people. By applying the natural anti-inflammatory and antimicrobial compounds found in aloe vera, you can minimize irritation and reduce the time spent recovering from poisonous plant exposure.

Scrapes

"Scrapes," "abrasions," and "scratches" all describe the same type of skin injury that results in a minimal, yet often painful, skin condition. While the skin is broken to an extent, the impact on the skin's layers is minimal with the affected area being contained to the outer layer, the epidermis. While many people have long regarded a scrape as a simple wound that doesn't require medical attention, it is important to note that germs, bacteria, and serious infections (even of the blood) can result from an unattended scrape.

In order to prevent infection and speed healing time, you can utilize aloe gel after cleaning the scrape, and continue applying aloe as often as desired until the wound is completely healed. Applying ample amounts of aloe to the site of a scrape and then bandaging it is the treatment method most often recommended; in doing so, you can safeguard the wound from environmental factors while improving the body's natural healing process.

Cuts

Cuts, lacerations, gashes, and tears all convey the same gruesome mental picture of a portion of skin that has been torn through the top layer of skin. Like burns, cuts can range in severity from requiring minimal medical attention to requiring stitches or sutures, but it is important to note that even the smallest of cuts and lacerations require thorough cleaning and treatment in order to prevent infection. Because the top layer of skin is cut, the body's subsequent layers of skin, bloodstream, and internal organs are all put at risk for infection.

Surprisingly, aloe vera has an added benefit for the treatment of cuts: with the immediate absorption of aloe into the skin, the aloe forms a water-tight seal at the wound's surface, contracting as it dries, sealing the wound shut, and serving as a protective barrier. Also providing anti-inflammatory agents, aloe acts to reduce the pain and swelling that can occur at the site of a cut or laceration.

Typically, a cut that is less than ¼" deep can be treated at home with these simple steps:

- **Stop the bleeding**—hold pressure until the body's clotting response commences.
- **Clean the wound**—rinse with clear water until the wound is free of dirt and debris (soap is not recommended in the cleaning of the wound because it may act as an irritant).
- **Apply an antibacterial, antiseptic, antimicrobial agent**—aloe vera delivers all the nutrients and phytochemicals necessary for the protection against infection, even of the most severe bacterial and viral varieties.
- **Bandage the wound**—by applying a bandage to the wound, you not only keep the wound protected from environmental factors, but also keep the aloe vera in place, undisturbed, for improved healing time and immunity protection.
- **Change dressing often**—bandages should be changed often (especially if wet or dirty) and reapplied after a new application of aloe has been administered to the cut.
- **Watch for signs of infection**—if the wound becomes red, swollen, irritated, painful, or hot, you should seek medical attention to ensure an infection has not spread to the surrounding area.

Bruises

Bruising occurs when trauma to the skin is harmful enough to break blood vessels, but without penetrating the skin. The broken blood vessels collect beneath the skin's surface, forming a blue, purple, green, or yellow bruise. The duration of a bruise is not just determined by the severity of the impact sustained, but also by the body's proficiency in cleansing the blood of dead or damaged cells.

Aloe vera can play an important part in speeding the recovery time of a bruise by delivering a number of helpful nutrients to the circulatory system and lymphatic system, assisting in the purging of the bruise's damaged cells. With a number of vitamins, minerals, and phytochemicals like vitamins A, C, and E, calcium, magnesium, zinc, and phenylalanine, aloe vera is able to deliver on-site repair of bruises. Its strong antioxidant and antiseptic agents cleanse the blood of the waste produced by the bruising.

Burns

Burns can occur from a variety of sources, but they are most commonly the result of an incident within the home. Whether the burn is minimal or severe, aloe vera has a number of powerful properties that act to promote healing, protect against infection, and produce the necessary skin cells for regeneration of the affected area. Classified into three categories, burns range in severity and result in health dangers specific to each category:

First-Degree Burns

First-degree burns are the most common type of burn and can result from a number of sources that range from unattended irons and excessively hot water to chemical and electrical sources. These burns affect the most superficial layer of skin and are characterized by redness of the affected area.

ESSENTIAL

Regardless of the cause of a burn, aloe vera can be used as an effective treatment not only after the burn occurs, but also throughout the recovery process. In the immediate treatment of a burn, aloe vera provides benefits that reduce pain and inflammation, while also preventing infection. Throughout the treatment, aloe vera can be administered to improve the recovery process by helping to deliver essential nutrients that can maximize healing and minimize healing time.

First-degree burns should be soaked in cold water for a minimum of 5 minutes and immediately treated with aloe vera. No ice or cotton should be applied to the site of the burn, as this will adversely affect the regeneration of new skin cells and inhibit the healing of the wound.

Second-Degree Burns

These burns generally result from an extended exposure to the source of the burn, allowing the subsequent layers of the skin to be affected. Because multiple layers of the skin are damaged, resulting in broken skin and an open wound, the risk of infection is much higher than with a first-degree burn in which the skin (while burned) stays intact. Blisters occur in a second-degree burn, which also increases the possibility of infection.

Immediately following a second-degree burn, the affected skin should be submerged in cold water for at least 15 minutes. The affected area should be treated with aloe vera immediately after soaking, and the burn should remain bandaged until the wound is healed. Treating the affected are with aloe not only helps the fibroblasts within the skin regenerate new skin cells, but the specific antimicrobial properties of aloe that help fend off infections caused by bacteria, viruses, and fungi safeguard the burn from possible environmental factors that thrive in open, moist wounds.

FACT

Aloe vera has long been known to be one of the most effective treatments for sunburn. Due to its lanolin content, aloe vera not only provides soothing nutrients that help reverse damage and discomfort resulting from sunburns, but also allows for deep penetration of these nutrients within the skin. In addition, aloe's antioxidants effectively combat the development of cancerous changes in cells, and the phytochemicals also help provide pain relief.

Third-Degree Burns

A third-degree burn is so severe that every layer of skin is destroyed. The nerves, blood, tissues, and even bones can be affected, and the possibility of developing a major infection of the blood as a result of the exposure is very high. Extreme blood loss and shock are common in third-degree burns, and with the nerves in the subsequent layers of skin destroyed, many victims of third-degree burns actually report minimal initial pain.

Calling 911 immediately after a third-degree burn occurs is crucial to the health and survival of the burn victim. It is essential that you not treat a third-degree burn at home; instead you should bring the burn victim to a hospital or qualified doctor. With the high risk of extreme conditions occurring throughout the body as a result of exposure from the skin's layers being completely destroyed, it is imperative that a third-degree burn victim seek medical attention as quickly as possible.

ALERT

By applying aloe to a burn, the natural healing properties of aloe can be used to minimize healing time and speed the regeneration of healthy skin cells. Before applying the aloe to the wound you should do a spot test on a healthy part of your skin to make sure your skin has no adverse reactions. Clean the affected wound well before applying the aloe vera, and maintain the health of the wound with proper wound care techniques such as changing bandages frequently.

Because of the increased risk to the blood posed by the skin's exposure to environmental elements, two common bacterial infections (sepsis and tetanus) are of great concern to victims of third-degree burns. As a powerful antiseptic, aloe vera has shown to be effective in cleaning the blood of bacteria, viruses, and microbes, minimizing the risk of the burn victim developing sepsis and tetanus. Aloe not only acts to protect the skin from microbe infiltration and the deadly internal infections that occur within the bloodstream, but it also provides the skin with the necessary properties that stimulate the protein synthesis of collagen and increase skin regeneration. Ask your doctor about using aloe on the burn and do not use it without your doctor's consent.

Insect Bites and Stings

Whether you're walking through the woods or sleeping soundly in your bed, an insect bite or sting can be an unexpected surprise with painful consequences. Ants, wasps, bees, spiders, and even caterpillars can inject venom through a bite or sting that can cause an irritation resulting in mild symptoms like itching and redness to severe symptoms such as damaged skin tissue and severe physical reactions. While the more severe reactions to bites and stings (such as difficulty breathing, vomiting, blurred vision, or severe swelling at the site of the bite or sting) require immediate medical attention, the common afflictions associated with insect bites can be quickly remedied with aloe vera.

FACT

Insect stings can deliver chemicals that not only cause pain and irritation, but can also result in inflammation that prolongs painful irritation for hours. By applying aloe vera to the site of a sting, the naturally occurring phytochemicals are able to combat the insect's poisons, reduce inflammation, and provide natural pain relief at the sight of the sting.

Acting as an antivenom, aloe vera provides a number of unique phytochemicals that quickly act to reduce the skin's reaction to an insect bite or sting by delivering their antihistamine, anti-inflammatory, and pain-relieving properties directly to the site of the bite or sting. With the added benefit of immunity-protecting antimicrobial, antiviral, and antibacterial properties, aloe vera can not only help relieve the pain of an insect bite, but also protect your skin from the risk of infection posed by itching, scratching, or environmental factors that introduce bacteria, viruses, and germs to a possibly open wound.

Irritations

The term *skin irritations* can include conditions of the skin that result in inflammation, redness, and discomfort. Rashes, eczema, dermatitis, rosacea, and even ringworm can all fall into this category. With a number of over-the-counter treatments that promise to provide relief for these conditions, a sufferer can easily be overwhelmed by the vast number of options available. Adding to the confusion is the lengthy list of chemicals and additives that are used in these products that may even misleadingly tote the phrase "all natural."

While these products may appear safe, they should be used with caution, as the ingredients may not have been sufficiently studied and can possibly contribute to a worsening of the original condition. In an effort to treat uncomfortable skin irritations that can be severe enough to interfere with daily life, consumers can opt for effective aloe vera rather than the mysterious additives in other products.

ALERT

Many illnesses and diseases can have side effects that adversely affect the skin. Dryness, inflammation, and underlying system dysfunction can create rashes, boils, irritations, and skin sensitivity. By ingesting aloe vera and applying aloe topically to skin irritations, it is possible to minimize not only the pre-existing conditions that contribute to skin conditions, but also the skin irritations that result.

With the ability to minimize the most common symptoms associated with skin irritations, aloe can be used as a treatment method safely and effectively. Aloe can provide temporary relief of the discomforts associated with skin irritations, and with its unique combination of vitamins, minerals, and phytochemicals, it can prevent these irritations from occurring or reoccurring.

Aloe has the ability to fend off bacteria, viruses, fungi, and germs that can aggravate the skin or weaken the immune system, making it susceptible to these common skin irritations. In addition to the germ-fighting properties, aloe also contains powerful anti-inflammatory agents that reduce the redness and swelling of the irritated area. Potent antioxidants help reduce the incidence of skin irritations from within the body by cleansing the body of illness- and irritation-promoting agents that can lead to the development or reoccurrence of skin irritations.

Serious Skin Conditions

From rosacea and psoriasis to shingles and severe inflammation, the serious conditions that can plague your skin are not only uncomfortable, but can be deadly. In treating the source of the issue, sometimes antibiotics are prescribed, and, more often than not, a host of other treatments are recommended. Oftentimes it is the skin that is one of the first areas of the body to show signs and symptoms of a more serious condition. In treating these serious skin issues internally as well as topically with aloe vera, you can utilize the naturally occurring elements of aloe in an effective treatment method that addresses both the internal causes and the resulting skin condition.

Rich in vitamins, minerals, and phytochemicals, aloe provides the body with an immediately usable form of powerful immunity-boosting aids. When you consume aloe in a liquid form, the aloe is immediately absorbed into the bloodstream, making each of its constituents available for use by every cell and organ in the body. Initially cleansing the blood with its antiseptic properties, the aloe vera sets into motion a disease-fighting attack on potentially harmful cellular changes with its antioxidant properties.

Since it contains large amounts of essential vitamins and minerals, aloe vera also starts to increase your body's supply of nutrients, making them available for use in a number of the body's processes immediately. While the blood, cells, and systems are receiving attention, the bacteria, viruses, and microbes in various areas of the body are killed, while anti-inflammatory properties begin to soothe areas of inflammation (even at the cellular level).

Topically, aloe vera begins the healing of bacterial, viral, or fungal-based conditions immediately by killing the source of the infection; this topical treatment is supported internally by the consumed aloe's cleansing effects on the blood and organ systems. With the added benefit of skin care provided by aloe, the topical treatment is also effective in reducing pain and inflammation at the site of skin conditions, while also providing protection from harmful changes within the cells of the skin.

Recipes

Bite Blaster

Bug bites can result in itchy, irritated areas of skin. And when you scratch the itchy skin, you risk introducing infection-causing bacteria to the area with every touch and scratch. The antimicrobial and anti-inflammatory agents contained in aloe and apple cider vinegar relieve inflammation and irritation while also preventing infection.

INGREDIENTS | MAKES ½ CUP

¼ cup aloe vera gel

¼ cup organic, unfiltered, and unpasteurized apple cider vinegar

1. Combine aloe vera and apple cider vinegar in a small bowl.

2. Soak a cotton ball with the solution and apply to the affected area as often as needed.

Sunburn Soother

Burns from prolonged sun exposure are not only uncomfortable, but can also result in harmful changes in the skin's cells. By using a combination of aloe vera, coconut oil, and vitamin E, you can moisturize and hydrate skin while applying powerful antioxidants that help safeguard the skin's health at a cellular level.

INGREDIENTS | MAKES 1 CUP

¼ cup aloe vera gel

½ cup coconut oil

¼ cup vitamin E oil

1. Combine ingredients in a glass jar and shake to combine well.

2. Apply solution to affected area as often as needed, until pain and redness subside.

Sweet Sting Remedy

*The discomfort of a bee or wasp sting can be remedied quickly and easily
with the soothing combination of aloe vera and honey. Packed with powerful antioxidants
that help fight uncomfortable inflammation, reduce pain, and protect against germs and
bacteria, this remedy can be quickly combined and applied to any sting for fast, effective relief.*

INGREDIENTS | MAKES ¼ CUP

2 tablespoons aloe vera gel

2 tablespoons pure organic honey

1. Combine aloe and honey in a blender and blend until completely emulsified.

2. Apply to the site of the sting, reapplying as often as necessary until pain and discomfort subsides.

Redness Reliever

The redness that appears on skin is a result of inflammation. Avenanthramides found in oats combine with the powerful anti-inflammatory and antimicrobial properties of aloe to relieve redness and reduce the inflammation causing it.

INGREDIENTS | MAKES 1 CUP

1 cup ground steel-cut oats

½ cup aloe vera gel

1. In a small bowl, combine oats and aloe and allow the oats to soak up the aloe completely, forming a paste.

2. Apply the paste to the affected area, covering with a moist towel or gauze.

3. Allow the paste to remain on the affected area for up to 30 minutes, repeating every 1–2 hours until redness subsides.

Healing Helper

Environmental agents, hormonal changes, or sun exposure can cause discoloration of the skin. Restorative collagen and elastin plus powerful antioxidants and phytochemicals replenish the skin's stores of essential nutrients to enhance the skin's healing process and naturally restore your skin's beauty.

INGREDIENTS | MAKES 2 CUPS

1½ cups pumpkin purée
½ cup coconut oil
½ cup aloe vera gel

1. In a medium bowl, combine all ingredients and blend by hand or with an immersion blender until well blended.

2. Apply the lotion to the affected area of skin and allow the lotion to set on the skin's surface for 10–15 minutes.

3. Repeat the process twice daily until discoloration subsides.

CHAPTER 5

Antiaging and Longevity

In the past, people thought that genetics alone dictated the length and quality of a person's life, but now we know that the choices you make countless times each day about your diet, exercise, sleep, and lifestyle can directly impact not only your health, energy level, and enthusiasm for life, but also the length of your life. To live a longer, healthier, more fulfilling life filled with enough energy, mental focus, and health to chase your dreams well into old age, aloe vera may be your key to the fountain of youth!

Energy and Stamina

The "midafternoon slump" that plagues most people at some point during the day is all too familiar to many of us. Low energy levels can negatively impact your day and place limitations on the activities in which you engage. This reduction in energy levels is one of the most common complaints of people as they age. But why does it happen? What process takes place in the body that slows energy production over the years, and more importantly, is it reversible?

FACT

Based on numerous studies on exercise recommendations for aging populations, most physicians now encourage people of all ages to engage in regular physical activity that increases the heart rate for at least 30 minutes, at least 3 days per week. This exercise recommendation has shown to reduce injuries, illnesses, and degeneration that are regularly associated with age.

Studies have identified a number of processes that contribute to the reduction in energy and stamina levels, which can be addressed and minimized with the addition of powerful nutrients—all of which can be provided by aloe vera. With a plethora of vitamins, minerals, and phytochemicals that combine to provide a variety of benefits, aloe vera supplies the body with specific components needed for healthy energy production that transcends age. Improving and maintaining cellular health, proper functioning of the organs, proper digestive functioning, and mental health are just a few examples of how the vitamins, minerals, and phytochemicals can provide antiaging benefits.

Energy is produced in the body through a number of synergistic processes that start with digestion and progress through several pathways the body uses to transform food and its nutrients into usable forms of energy. Nutrient deficiencies can cause fatigue because a deficiency in just one of the major energy-producing elements can not only impair energy production, but also impede the processes of the body's systems as a whole. Because these processes need essential nutrients in order to function properly, it is absolutely imperative that a focus is placed on quality nutrition as you age. In particular, there are three deficiencies in the diet that can contribute to reduction in energy levels as you age: B vitamins, magnesium, and antioxidants.

B Vitamins

B vitamins play a crucial role in the production of energy. Mitochondria, which are responsible for converting food into energy, rely heavily on vitamins from food for use in a number of biochemical reactions that contribute to energy production. A diet deficient in B vitamins adversely impacts the mitochondrial production of energy. A vitamin B deficiency also contributes to reduced efficiency in other processes that contribute to energy production, including oxygen delivery among red blood cells, communication between the central nerve system and peripheral nerve system through nerve cells, and the development of serotonin and dopamine in the brain.

ESSENTIAL

With regular physical activity the body is able to engage in activity far more easily than without regular activity. By simply engaging in various activities that require different ranges of motion and that increase the heart rate to different levels for varying periods of time, the body is able to function properly in a number of situations, allowing for improved performance, results, and benefits.

The body's systems that contribute to the production and availability of energy in the body all rely on an adequate intake of B vitamins. Restoring the body's supply of B_1 (thiamine), B_2 (riboflavin), B_3 (niacin), B_5 (pantothenic acid), B_6 (pyridoxine), B_7 (biotin), B_9 (folic acid), and B_{12} (cyanocobalamin) is essential for optimum energy production, This can easily be done with a simple serving of 25 ml of aloe vera three times daily.

Magnesium

An essential mineral that is involved in up to 300 metabolic reactions in the body, magnesium plays a major role in energy production. Magnesium is used by the mitochondria in the formation and storage of the energy molecule ATP (adenosine triphosphate). Deficiencies in magnesium adversely affect the production of energy by the mitochondria by weakening the cell's "powerhouse" and reducing its ability to fight free radical damage, leaving it open to oxidative stress. A surprising 23 percent of Americans are believed to be deficient in magnesium. As you age, it's important to consider magnesium deficiency as a possible contributor to fatigue. The same 25 ml serving of aloe that resolves B vitamin deficiencies also provides the magnesium your body needs.

Antioxidants

Antioxidants are naturally occurring compounds that neutralize free radicals by preventing oxygen from reacting with other compounds that can result in harmful changes. Antioxidants protect the mitochondria from becoming damaged, which could reduce energy output. By improving the mitochondrial defenses of the cells, antioxidants safeguard the energy levels of the entire body. Aloe vera contains a variety of nutrients and phytochemicals, such as vitamins A, C, and E, and anthraquinones, which promote antioxidant activity within the cells. These substances have been shown to increase the protection of the mitochondria, as well as a number of other cellular components that contribute to proper system functioning.

Immunity

Maintaining a powerful immune system is absolutely essential in the pursuit of a long, healthy life. Vitamins, minerals, and antioxidants supply the body with the essentials needed to function properly and protect the body from infection and disease. Even with ample amounts of vitamins and nutrients available through the diet, the body can succumb to illness or infection when just one of the essential nutrients is deficient. By supplementing your diet with aloe vera, you can ensure your body has the nutrients it needs and also provide it with the added benefits of improved protection from aloe vera's phytochemicals. Aloe vera's anthraquinones help fight inflammation and illness and safeguard your health in a number of ways:

- **Inflammation:** You're probably familiar with inflammation occurring in various parts of the body—where skin has become irritated or infected, in arthritic joints, or at the site of an injury. But inflammation also can take place at the cellular levels at any point in the body. This internal, "silent" inflammation can result in dangerous changes that can interfere with proper functioning or cause cells to mutate. Inflammation can be minimized with aloe vera's unique blend of plant sterols, campesterol, beta-sitosterol, and lupeol.
- **Illness:** With powerful defenses against bacteria, viruses, fungi, and microbes, the anthraquinones of aloe combat illnesses and help improve immunity against future illnesses.
- **Protection:** The saponins of aloe vera cleanse the circulatory system while counteracting the effects of cancerous elements. The saponins are supported by the antioxidant activity provided by vitamins C and E.

Cognitive Function

As you age, your cognitive health can decline in a number of ways, most commonly manifesting in reduced memory capacity. The best way to minimize the effects of aging on cognitive abilities is to work to prevent them in the first place.

Aloe vera provides your body with phytochemicals and nutrients that can assist in each of the recommended areas of focus for maintaining brain health. Through a number of effective applications that involve diet, exercise, sleep, and improved mental functioning techniques, you can help safeguard your brain from some of the effects of aging. Aloe vera can provide a number of helpful benefits in this area.

Diet

Every single biochemical reaction that occurs in the body depends upon nutrients like vitamins, minerals, amino acids, and enzymes obtained through the diet. It's absolutely essential to consume a clean, wholesome diet in order to maintain optimal cognitive abilities. A lack of quality nutrition can result in symptoms like low energy levels, an inability to focus on tasks, and a lack of mental clarity. Aloe vera promotes quality brain functioning with ample amounts of vitamins, minerals, and phytochemicals that assist in nerve functioning, cell health, and blood clarity.

Exercise

Exercise doesn't only benefit the body. Your mood benefits from the production of endorphins and hormones in the brain. Exercise also improves mental functioning by stimulating the senses that provide information to the brain, activating muscles and nerves that communicate with the brain, and improving blood flow to all the body's organs, all of which help maintain mental vigor. All these processes are enhanced with the use of aloe vera because the amino acids in aloe assist in the production of hormones and enzymes required by the brain to process the information of biofeedback and the physical actions and stimulation of exercise. With adequate exercise performed for just 30 minutes three times per week in combination with daily servings of aloe vera, you can improve your brain functioning while also benefiting your body.

ESSENTIAL

When you engage in physical activity, your body is put into motion, making your brain responsible for interpreting multiple messages from all the body's senses and systems simultaneously. Through paying attention to other participants, a ball's direction, and hand-eye coordination—all while avoiding obstacles—the brain is exercised anytime the body is!

Sleep

While most people regard sleep as a time of rest, the brain uses these precious hours of shuteye for regeneration and preparation. The most widely accepted recommendation for sleep is 6–8 hours nightly. With just one night of reduced sleep, the brain reacts with slower reaction time, reduced focus, impaired attention span, and a number of additional physical symptoms. Aloe vera contains nutrients and phytochemicals that help minimize factors that inhibit quality sleep, like anxiety, digestive issues, and physical pain.

Aloe also contains tryptophan, which can help the body achieve a longer, more restful period of sleep.

Mental Functioning Techniques

In the same way that the muscles atrophy and die without use, the brain can quickly degenerate and develop processing issues as a result of lack of stimulation. With "brain games," meditation, and stimulation such as reading and activity, the brain can remain spry and active, just as physical fitness allows the muscles to do the same.

Aloe vera's nutrients help improve energy levels during activity and also produce a calming effect during times of relaxation and focus. Aloe helps the brain to be vivacious and alert when need be, while also being able to sufficiently enjoy the restorative times of focus, clarity, and calm and relaxation that can be just as beneficial.

Bone and Muscle Maintenance

Without adequate amounts of the vitamins, minerals, enzymes, amino acids, and phytochemicals the body needs, a deficiency develops. Deficiencies in any of the necessary nutrients are remedied naturally by the body by extracting the nutrients from concentrated sources in the body.

ALERT

Be sure to vary your exercise routine. By alternating types of activity to focus on various aspects of the body's ability and functioning, you can improve your overall health exponentially. Alternate cardiovascular exercise, strength-training exercises, and flexibility training, and your body and its systems will benefit from various challenges placed upon it when engaged in different activities.

For example, if your body is deficient in calcium, it will use calcium stored in bones and teeth to meet its needs. The same process is utilized when the body requires more protein than is being consumed in the diet. The body turns to the most concentrated available source of protein—the muscles—for its needs, and slowly degrades the muscles in order to provide systems with adequate amounts of the essential building blocks needed.

Aloe vera is able to provide the body with ample amounts of the vitamins and minerals the body needs in order to promote and maintain the health of the body's structural components, while also improving the body's ability to absorb these essential nutrients.

Bone Health

Throughout the younger years of life, the body builds bone mass and develops density that peaks at around age thirty. Once the body reaches the stopping point of bone development, it's important to focus on maintaining the bone density you have. As the years progress past the age of thirty, your diet is the primary source of the vitamins and minerals used by the body to prevent bone loss.

If the body becomes deficient in essential nutrients, the stores of those nutrients become the source the body depends on. For those who are deficient in calcium and magnesium, this can spell disaster for bone health, because the body turns to the bones and teeth for their concentrated calcium and magnesium stores. The result is a gradual degradation of the bones' density, which can in turn contribute to conditions like osteoporosis.

Providing B vitamins, vitamin C, vitamin E, and many minerals required in the promotion of bone health, aloe vera acts to reduce the incidence of bone issues associated with age by assisting in mineral absorption.

FACT

Aloe vera not only contributes a number of vitamins and minerals that are essential in maintaining bone health, but also improves the body's ability to absorb and store these essential nutrients within the bone. These benefits contribute to the structural support of bones and can also reduce the chances of degradation in bone mass resulting from common deficiencies later in life.

The vitamins C and E that are found in the aloe vera leaf help improve the absorption of minerals consumed in the diet, making them more readily bioavailable for storage and utilization in the processes associated in bone development. This improved absorption also ensures the proper provision of the bone-building essentials to the body's systems and processes that also require adequate supply, reducing the chance of deficiencies that result in the body's dependence on the bones as stores of the nutrients.

Combined with a quality diet that contributes ample amounts of calcium by way of leafy greens and vegetables, 25 ml of aloe vera three times daily can help improve bone health, keeping you strong and protected throughout your later years.

Muscle Maintenance

Building muscle is a science, requiring a number of macronutrients, micronutrients, and supporting lifestyle factors such as adequate exercise and sleep. The process of building and maintaining quality muscle stores is one that provides health and vitality throughout your life.

QUESTION

Is muscle loss an inevitable result of aging?
As you age, your body undergoes a number of processes that pose challenges in developing muscle mass and maintaining muscle mass. With a diet rich in proteins and complex carbohydrates, physical activity, and regular aloe vera consumption, anybody can help fight muscle loss and maintain adequate muscle mass throughout life.

Muscles provide structural support, provide the body with stores of the essential building blocks of life (protein), and ensure the proper processing and utilization of a number of nutrients for use throughout the body. If you don't maintain adequate muscle mass as you age, you fatigue quickly, your strength declines, your abilities become limited, and all the body's systems that depend on the structure of muscles begin to suffer. While this degeneration sounds like the "normal aging process," it doesn't have to be. With aloe vera and a diet of clean, whole foods that provide ample amounts of nutrients, you can maintain dense muscle mass that will help keep you strong throughout your life.

Aloe vera can help improve your body's overall composition while assisting in the process of muscle maintenance by contributing a number of powerful components to your daily diet, like electrolytes, glycogen, and amino acids:

- **Electrolytes:** charged ions that when mixed with water improve performance of the muscles during activity, and are lost through the body's sweat. Electrolytes, including sodium, potassium, magnesium, calcium, and chloride, are essential in maintaining adequate muscle composition, and can all be found in aloe vera.
- **Glycogen:** a source of energy that is stored by the body in the muscles for use during activity. It is developed through the consumption of complex carbohydrates supplied by whole foods such as fruit and vegetables, as well as aloe vera.
- **Amino acids:** the muscular system requires amino acids and protein in order to build, maintain, and repair muscle tissue. Providing an astounding twenty of the twenty-two amino acids necessary for proper muscle maintenance, aloe vera has been identified as a great source of this muscle-maintaining element.

While these nutrients are often found in plentiful amounts in healthy foods, they can be minimized by deficiencies in other areas of the diet that impede their absorption or utilization. Consuming a minimum of 25 ml of aloe vera up to three times daily can improve your body's functioning, your energy levels, and your energy output, helping you maintain adequate muscle mass for years to come.

Recipes

Energy Essential Smoothie

This smoothie provides ample protein, carbohydrates, and antioxidants to keep you energized for hours! Blueberries provide powerful antioxidants, and aloe supports the body's ability to break down complex carbohydrates and proteins while providing a number of vital amino acids.

INGREDIENTS | SERVES 1

¼ cup aloe vera juice

½ cup frozen blueberries

1 cup unsweetened vanilla almond milk

Combine all ingredients in a blender. Blend until smooth.

Sweet Stamina Smoothie

This combination of vibrant produce provides ample amounts of essential nutrients that are needed for steady energy levels throughout the day. This refreshing smoothie provides you with vitamins, minerals, and antioxidants, along with phytochemicals to improve the body's absorption and utilization of the nutrients.

INGREDIENTS | SERVES 2

¼ cup aloe vera juice
2½ cups brewed green tea, chilled
1 large kale leaf
½ medium apple, peeled and cored
½ medium pear, peeled and cored

Combine all ingredients in a blender. Blend until smooth.

Creamy Raspberry Omega Smoothie

The nutrients provided by the antioxidant-rich aloe vera, vitamin C–packed raspberries, omega-rich flaxseeds, and probiotic yogurt combine to promote immunity and brain health and improve the functioning of the cardiovascular and digestive systems.

INGREDIENTS | SERVES 1

¼ cup aloe vera juice

½ cup plain Greek yogurt

½ cup frozen raspberries

⅛ cup ground flaxseed

¼ cup water

1. Combine all ingredients except water in a blender.

2. Blend until smooth, adding water as needed until desired consistency is achieved.

Strawberries and Cream Smoothie

This simple smoothie can be a bone-building breakfast or scrumptious snack that leaves your bones, brain, and body satisfied and strong. Maple syrup adds sweetness and antioxidants.

INGREDIENTS | SERVES 2

¼ cup aloe vera juice

1 cup plain Greek yogurt

½ cup frozen strawberries

¼ cup peeled and sliced cucumber

1 tablespoon organic maple syrup

Combine all ingredients in a blender. Blend until smooth.

Perfect Protein

Protein and amino acids help your muscles remain strong,
boosting your benefits from activity and helping you maintain overall health year after year!

INGREDIENTS | SERVES 2

¼ cup aloe vera juice

1½ cups unsweetened almond milk

½ cup almonds

½ cup pitted chopped dates

1. Combine aloe vera, almond milk, and almonds in a blender and blend until almonds are completely emulsified.

2. Add dates and blend until smooth.

CHAPTER 6

Beauty Treatments

Take a quick glance down the beauty aisle of any department store and you'll see that the desire for improved beauty is being met with countless products available to treat every area of your body from your hair and face to your skin and feet. Unlike these new or fad beauty treatments, the first recorded applications of aloe were those of Cleopatra and Nefertiti, who utilized the benefits of aloe to improve the beauty of their hair and skin. With the information available about aloe today, we know that aloe's aesthetic benefits go far beyond skin and hair, and can also be used to improve the appearance of your teeth, nails, and even your eyes!

Skin

Your skin is a direct reflection of the internal and external condition of your body. When there is an upset in the biochemical reactions taking place in any of your body's systems, your skin is the first place that those upsets are apparent. Taking only a matter of 2–4 days to show the effects of your hygiene, diet, sleep regimen, and exercise routine, your skin accurately portrays the condition of your body in a number of ways. Discoloration, wrinkles, sagging, oily or dry conditions, acne, and even cellulite can all result from the lack of attention to any number of factors that are essential in caring for your skin and optimizing its appearance. Luckily, studies have shown that a number of nutrients and biochemical reactions are responsible for the physical effects on skin, allowing you to improve your overall health through a variety of dietary and lifestyle choices.

With aloe vera, you can improve the health and appearance of your skin in a number of ways. Topically, the results can be seen immediately, increasing over the course of its use. By applying the aloe directly to the surface of your skin, the potent nutrients contained within the aloe are able to penetrate the skin's surface, providing benefits externally as well as to the unseen layers that support the external layers. This process results in firmer, less blemished skin that is able to refute naturally occurring damage from the sun and environmental exposures. Knowing that the skin's regeneration process is constant, it seems obvious that you should take great care of the soon-to-be-seen supportive layers of new skin as you tend to the external layers.

FACT

Harsh chemicals that negatively affect the quality of your hair, nails, and skin health can be found almost everywhere. Between cleaning products, beauty products, and even prolonged exposure to seemingly harmless solutions, these degrading elements can adversely affect the health of the systems that directly promote the growth and well-being of the hair, skin, and nails. By being aware of the environmental elements that can wreak havoc on beauty, you can safeguard your overall health and maintain your natural beauty.

The benefits of aloe to the skin are not limited to topical applications. Ingesting aloe vera allows the potent nutrients to explore the body, remedying the upsets that can occur at any point from the bloodstream to your digestive functioning and metabolism levels. It is easy to understand how aloe vera can be utilized to promote the healthiest appearance of your skin through the vitamins and minerals that are found in it. In addition to providing these nutrients directly, the aloe affects the body's ability to absorb and utilize the nutrients, not only improving the skin but also improving the body's overall health and optimal functioning, which also promotes skin health indirectly!

Vitamins

The most important vitamins required by the skin for optimal health have been identified as being A, C, E, B complex, and K. While each of these vitamins plays an important part in the skin's health, it is worth mentioning that the benefits to the skin are not only direct, but also indirect in that these nutrients provide support to a number of the body's systems and processes that indirectly benefit the skin by maintaining proper blood flow, optimum digestion, healthy immunity, etc.

- **Vitamin A:** essential in the development and repair of skin tissue, vitamin A (also referred to as beta-carotene) can improve your body's production of essential skin cells that can contribute to a reduction in skin conditions (such as eczema and psoriasis), reduce the incidence of fine lines and wrinkles on your face, and may minimize discoloration.
- **Vitamins C and E:** the *Journal of Investigative Dermatology* has long promoted the use of vitamins C and E for their effects in preventing sunburns and minimizing the catastrophic damage to DNA that results from extended periods of sun exposure. Improving the health of skin cells and maximizing their ability to prevent damage, vitamins C and E have shown to be effective antioxidants that can be utilized topically and externally. Aloe vera has shown in numerous studies to improve the bioavailability of vitamins C and E, while also improving the body's ability to absorb and utilize the vitamins.
- **Vitamin K:** more widely accepted as the vitamin responsible for improving blood content and its ability to clot, it may seem surprising to include

vitamin K in this list, but its effect on the blood is exactly why it's here. Vitamin K has been shown to have surprising results on bruises, under-eye circles, and even wrinkles by improving the circulation and blood flow. With the added benefit of improving your skin's glow as a result of the improved circulation, vitamin K is an absolute essential in the improved appearance of your skin.

- **B vitamins:** Biotin is one of the best-known B vitamins, and it is one of the most valuable when it comes to the condition of your skin. Biotin helps maintain the skin's elasticity and keeps the skin's surface adequately hydrated, making it beneficial to any skin prone to dryness or aging. Niacin is another B vitamin that promotes the health of your skin, and it does so by acting as a powerful anti-inflammatory that can fight redness, irritation, and even acne.

With all of these essential vitamins found in aloe vera, normal consumption of this astounding product contributes to the improvement of health and wellness in a number of ways!

FACT

Retinol is actually a form of vitamin A. Found in a number of effective skin creams, retinol-a has been proven to reduce the incidence of acne and eczema while improving wrinkles and discoloration.

Minerals

Traditionally thought of as supporting blocks of structure in the human body, minerals actually play an essential part in maintaining healthy skin through their ability to provide protection, regeneration, and maintenance of skin cells. The minerals selenium, copper, and zinc are imperative to skin health.

- **Selenium:** a rarely mentioned mineral, selenium has been identified as playing a major role in the prevention of skin cancer. According to the American Medical Association, selenium is effective in preventing skin issues resulting from sun exposure. Selenium has been shown to reduce skin cancers by up to 37 percent and reduce the number of deaths related to skin cancer by up to 50 percent! Two hundred micrograms per day is the generally accepted recommendation for daily selenium intake.

- **Copper and zinc:** by joining forces with vitamin C and zinc, copper helps form elastin, the skin structure composed of fibers beneath the skin that gives skin even tone and elasticity. While working synergistically with copper to provide skin's elasticity, zinc regulates oil production on the skin's surface, helping to reduce the incidence of acne.

Luckily, all of these essential minerals are found in aloe, and contribute each of their amazing benefits to some extent.

Amino Acids

Aloe contains a staggering twenty of the twenty-two amino acids the body needs to function. With many of these amino acids producing powerful antioxidant effects in the body, it is no surprise that there are three amino acids that play critical roles in the skin's health and preservation of the skin's beauty. Glycine, proline, and lysine combine to promote the body's production of collagen. In improving collagen production, these amino acids directly benefit the skin by minimizing the appearance of fine lines and wrinkles, while also improving the production of renewed skin cells that can replace damaged or adversely affected cells. With the rich amount of amino acids contained in every dose of aloe vera, all of these benefits can be enjoyed by the avid aloe vera consumer!

Hair

When it comes to hair, the amount of time and money people are willing to spend is nothing short of shocking. Trillions of dollars are spent on hair care, and it can be startling to realize that much of this money is focused on products and treatments that actually cause more harm than good.

The hair is a reflection of the health of the body presently as well as up to 2–6 months prior. Knowing this, you can better understand why those months of illness or haphazard dieting resulted in lackluster hair that showed the lack of nutrients and healthy function your body experienced.

As with all the areas of beauty covered here, the components of diet, exercise, and lifestyle choices play a major role in the condition of your hair, contributing to its health or degrading the main components of your body that promote its health. With aloe, though, you can improve your body's overall health and watch the difference in your hair as you use it topically as well as internally.

With aloe vera providing amino acids (the building blocks of protein); vitamins B, C, and E; and the minerals iron, selenium, copper, and magnesium, this all-natural beauty treatment improves the look of your hair through topical use and improves the health of your hair as it grows through internal benefits. Whether you utilize aloe vera for hair benefits through topical applications, or include the potent product in your daily smoothies, snacks, and meals, the daily use of aloe vera can provide a wide range of benefits to every strand! With daily use, many people notice results within a matter of weeks; increasing the effectiveness of the aloe vera's benefits to the hair, topical and ingested uses are suggested. These essential nutrients synergistically work to develop hair, maintain its strength, and produce the color, texture, and condition of each and every strand. With just one of the elements in short supply, the result can be weak and brittle hair that is prone to breakage, slow growth, thinning strands, or even hair loss.

As with all the body's processes and the connections between those processes, poor system function in just one area of the body can wreak havoc on hair and its quality. To improve the health of your hair, you should focus on using aloe not only for its direct benefits to your locks, but also for its benefits to the systems that promote healthy hair growth. The three main areas of concern regarding the health of your hair are the circulatory system, the production of protein, and the nutrient density of your diet. Aloe vera has a profound impact on hair health by not only providing support in each of these three areas but also by promoting overall body health.

The Circulatory System

With improved circulation, your scalp receives the necessary blood flow that delivers nutrients, stimulates hair growth, and improves the health of your hair's strands. Aloe vera's cleansing effect on the blood improves the metabolic functions of the body, helping the circulatory system run more efficiently and ultimately improving the appearance of your hair. Aloe vera can also help the circulatory system process iron, an essential hair nutrient, by not only supplying it, but also by improving the amount of iron that is absorbed from the diet and utilized by the blood and the body.

Protein Production

Your hair is created using a specialized protein in the body called keratin. As with all proteins, amino acids play a major role in keratin production and utilization. Without proper amounts of amino acids in the body, protein production and utilization suffers, as do your strands. Aloe vera provides healthy doses of twenty of the twenty-two amino acids essential for proteins needed throughout the body (including keratin) for healthy hair development and growth.

ESSENTIAL

The amount of protein in your diet directly affects every aspect of beauty. With adequate supplies of all amino acids necessary for the body to promote the health and well-being of skin, hair, nails, teeth, and eyes, it is absolutely imperative to include ample amounts of clean protein like chicken, fish, and low-fat meats in your daily diet. By including aloe vera in your daily routine, you can ensure the body's requirements for amino acids are met *and* that the body is better able to absorb and utilize each and every one.

Diet

When your diet is limited in terms of calories or nutrients, the results can be catastrophic. Because each of your body's systems require ample amounts of specific nutrients, a depletion in any one can result in poor system functioning. Where one system fails to function, many others are affected, and the result is similar to cascading dominos—and your hair may be one of the casualties.

If you focus your diet on colorful whole foods like fruit and vegetables that are packed with vitamins A, C, and E, you can ensure your body is getting the adequate supplies of the nutrients it needs to thrive. For maximum benefits, including aloe vera in your daily diet will not only supply added vitamins, minerals, and phytochemicals, but it will supplement those your diet may be lacking while also improving your body's absorption and utilization of those your body needs to thrive. This will be apparent in your overall health, as well your hair.

Teeth

From braces to teeth whitening, a winning smile can now be bought, but at a pretty high purchase price. Aside from dental aesthetics, the root (no pun intended) of many dental visits stems from problematic issues that could have easily been prevented with proper care. Whether the goal is to keep a child's teeth cavity-free, an adult's smile free of coffee stains, or an elderly person's mouth free of dental disease, the same rules apply: Prevention is the best medicine.

In terms of oral care, the most important areas that affect oral health are the bacteria and microbe levels of the mouth, the nutrients that promote healthy teeth and gums, inflammation, and pH balance. With these factors all contributing to the health and appearance of teeth, it is imperative that special care be taken to meet each need for optimum oral health. Not surprisingly, aloe vera is able to improve the health of the mouth and the appearance of the teeth by maximizing the benefits and minimizing threats.

Improved Immunity

In order to maintain a healthy smile, an optimal balance of bacteria and microbes in the mouth must be maintained. Ever-present microbes and bacteria in the mouth are necessary to break down food and prepare it for digestion, produce saliva, etc. When the bacteria that form plaque or the microbes that contribute to, or result from, breeding illnesses invade the mouth, problems and issues can occur. While brushing and flossing regularly to remove infectious elements is recommended, you can also use aloe vera as an effective antibacterial, antiviral, antimicrobial, and antiseptic agent that can help reduce the incidence of illness while safely maintaining the "good" bacteria and microbes that maintain oral health. A simple swishing of aloe vera every time you brush your teeth, or three times per day, can provide protection and prevention!

ALERT

When people think of calcium deficiency, most have immediate thoughts relating to bone health, but oral health relies on adequate supplies of these basic minerals just as much. Aloe vera is able to ensure that every aspect of oral health remains intact by promoting absorption of key minerals and providing supporting nutrients that help in the maintenance of teeth and gums, and even combat digestive disorders commonly associated with unhealthy oral conditions.

Adequate Nutrition

When your body suffers from deficiencies in protein, calcium, phosphorous, zinc, iron, vitamin A, vitamin C, or B vitamins, your oral health can suffer with weakened tooth structure or gum disease. These consequences can be easily avoided with the implementation of aloe vera. Rich in each of the vitamins and minerals necessary for oral health, aloe vera can assist in the absorption of the valuable nutrients your mouth needs to maintain healthy teeth and gums.

Inflammation

Inflammation of the gums is not only uncomfortable, but the condition can also lead to a number of serious issues that plague the mouth and the entire body. With inflammation of the gums comes a disastrous combination of unhealthy cell growth, red and irritated gums, exposed teeth roots, and increased saliva production that expedites the delivery of the unhealthy elements to the bloodstream and body. With aloe vera's powerful anti-inflammatory and antiseptic agents, the gums are able to return to their original condition preinflammation while the antiseptic properties provide protection against disease at the site of the inflammation as well as throughout the body.

pH Balance

Long known for its ability to return pH balance to the body, aloe vera has been shown to reduce the incidence of improper pH in the mouth as well. An unbalanced pH balance of the saliva is most commonly found in diabetes patients due to high blood sugar, but an unhealthy pH can result from a number of health issues, and it can become a precursor to dangerous oral health conditions. With its provision of arginine, an important amino acid, aloe vera is able to restore the pH balance of the mouth to healthy levels while also reducing the incidence of cavities.

Nails

As with your skin, hair, and teeth, your nails provide a pretty good insight into your overall quality of health. The quality of your diet and lifestyle directly affect the condition of your nails and dictate their strength, length, and rate of growth. If you find yourself suffering from weak, brittle nails that rarely reach a desirable length, often grow in a haphazard manner, develop areas of discoloration in the nail bed, or are surrounded by red and irritated cuticles, these may be signs of underlying health issues that need addressing. Because your nails' condition can be a result of weeks of care or neglect, identifying possible issues and areas of improvement can be quite easy, allowing you to make the appropriate changes and see results in as little as 1–4 weeks.

The nails are composed of stratified epithelium. Epithelial cells are what make up the skin, and the nails are only different from the skin in that the nails are composed of multiple layers of epithelial with the added keratin proteins that provide the hardness for protection and growth. With a similar composition to skin, your nails require a similar nutrient combination that contains protein, vitamins, and minerals, as well as protection from infections that can often wreak havoc on the delicate epithelial cells.

Lifestyle factors such as sleep, exercise, and diet require the most attention if strong, healthy nails are what you desire. Not surprisingly, the benefits aloe vera can have on the health of your nails are quite impressive. With the addition of aloe vera to your daily diet, you can effectively improve your overall health in just a matter of weeks . . . with the added benefit of beautiful nails!

ESSENTIAL

Many issues relating to digestion can actually interfere with the absorption of essential nutrients needed for the proper maintenance of the very building blocks needed for healthy skin, hair, nails, eyes, and teeth. By focusing a diet on nutrient-rich foods, and including aloe vera in your daily diet, you can improve digestion and minimize the incidence of digestive disorders that can interfere with the absorption and usage of the very nutrients your body needs.

Diet

With a diet focused on clean, whole foods, you can improve your daily consumption of vitamins, minerals, and naturally occurring phytochemicals. Fruit and vegetables provide your body with a boost of these essentials, and with the addition of aloe vera, your benefits increase even more!

With a host of necessary nutrients for nail growth like the vitamins A, C, E, as well as a variety of B vitamins, plus iron, zinc, and magnesium, and the added benefit of amino acids that play a major part in the production of keratin, aloe vera not only provides your body's systems that support nail health with the must-have's for proper functioning, but it also directly promotes the healthy growth and maintenance of your nails. Minimizing the incidence of deficiencies that can result in brittleness, white spots, and horizontal ridges, aloe vera acts as the super supplement that contains everything your nails need, and more!

Exercise

The importance of proper blood circulation can never be emphasized too much. Providing the entire body with the blood, cells, nourishment, nutrients, enzymes, and reactions it needs to function properly, the circulatory system is (literally!) the heartbeat that keeps the body in motion. Without the proper circulation to your hands and feet, the effects on the health of your nails can be catastrophic. Exercise helps improve the body's circulation. With just three to five 30-minute bouts of exercise each week, you can improve your body's circulatory system function.

Aloe vera also provides a number of blood-cleansing properties that keep the circulatory system free of health issues that can slow the pumping of blood, reduce energy levels, and increase the incidence of illness and disease. With ample amounts of aloe vera in your diet, you can maintain a healthy circulatory system and a high energy level so you can maintain the exercise regimen that improves the health of your nails.

FACT

Internally and externally, aloe vera is able to improve the appearance and health of nails. By supplying nutrients to the body and all of the body's systems that are involved in nail growth, ingesting aloe vera helps in the improvement and maintenance of nails from the inside-out! Externally, topical applications of aloe to the nails, such as soaking, help to support and protect the growth and health of nails directly at the source!

Protection

Because the nails are composed of delicate tissue, and because the hands are exposed to more germs and illness-producing microbes than any other part of the body, it is absolutely essential that you take care to keep your hands free of germs, bacteria, viruses, and fungi. Washing your hands with soap and water often throughout the day can improve the health of your hands and reduce the incidence of infection, but aloe vera can also assist in the prevention of illnesses by providing its anthraquinones throughout the bloodstream and directly on the nails and hands. These powerful phytochemicals not only combat bacteria, viruses, and germs, but also prevent the fungal infections that can plague nail beds and cuticles. Improving the ability of your hands to retain moisture while also improving the protection against infection makes aloe vera the only natural nail-promoting essential you need! Through regular topical applications of aloe to the skin's surface, such as smoothing the aloe vera gel onto hands like a lotion or soaking nails in the aloe vera liquid, you can maximize the benefits that are all ready being produced through the regular consumption of the aloe vera liquid.

Lifestyle Factors

The two lifestyle factors that contribute to damaged nails more than others are smoking and consistently exposing your nails and hands to moisture. Because smoking exposes your nails directly to the site of the burning cigarette's off-gasses as well as the inhaled and exhaled resulting smoke, the nails develop stains and damage from the tar and hazardous materials found within the smoke and the cigarette itself. Refraining from smoking benefits your entire body and will help keep your nails beautiful and free of tar stains.

Excessive exposure to moisture may sound like a condition limited to dishwashers and people in the detailing industry, but think about how often you wash your hands throughout the day, submerge your hands in water, shower, bathe, brush your teeth, etc. Each and every time your hands are exposed to water, the nails become soft and can more easily succumb to infection. In order to prevent this from happening, a simple pair of dishwashing gloves can be used for chores, and special care during and after exposure should be taken.

Recipes

Awesome Eyes Smoothie

This smoothie provides eyes with protection against illness and disease while maintaining natural health. With a number of vitamins, minerals, and antioxidants that promote eye health and appearance, the benefits of aloe vera maximize the eyes' beauty and health!

INGREDIENTS | SERVES 2

¼ cup aloe vera juice

1 large sweet potato, baked or steamed and skin removed

1 tablespoon ground flaxseed

2 cups unsweetened almond milk

1 teaspoon ground cinnamon

Combine all ingredients in a blender. Blend until smooth.

Oily Skin Saving Mask

With nutrients, enzymes, and citric acid, these ingredients minimize oil and associated irritations by providing precisely what oily skin needs to return to a natural, healthy balance. Aloe increases nutrient absorption into the skin.

INGREDIENTS | MAKES ENOUGH FOR 4 APPLICATIONS

¼ cup aloe vera gel

¼ cup coconut oil

1 tablespoon lemon juice

1 tablespoon organic, unfiltered, and unpasteurized apple cider vinegar

1 cup white or brown sugar

1. Combine aloe vera, coconut oil, lemon juice, and apple cider vinegar in a blender, and blend until ingredients are thoroughly combined.

2. Add sugar and blend for 2 seconds.

3. Apply ⅛ cup of solution to the face, allowing it to set for 10 minutes before rinsing.

4. Store remaining solution in an airtight container in a cool, dark place. Blend again before next use.

Sensitive Skin Soother

Sensitive skin is easily irritated and sometimes painful. This all-natural aloe treatment can be applied to any area of the body to provide relief from irritations, illness, or simply sensitivity.

INGREDIENTS | MAKES ENOUGH FOR 6 APPLICATIONS

¼ cup aloe vera gel

¼ cup coconut oil

⅛ cup pure organic honey

¼ cup vitamin E oil

1. Place all ingredients in a blender and blend until thoroughly combined.

2. Apply ⅛ cup of solution to the face, allowing it to set for 10 minutes before rinsing.

3. Store remaining solution in an airtight container in a cool, dark place. Blend again before next use.

Happy Hair Soak

Dull, dry hair can be prone to frizz and breakage. But this protein-rich conditioning treatment provides hair with restorative health-promoting essentials that help every strand absorb the exact nutrients needed to be soft, shiny, and beautiful.

INGREDIENTS | MAKES ENOUGH FOR 1 TREATMENT

¼ cup aloe vera gel
1 cup unsweetened almond milk
¼ cup vitamin E oil
2–4 drops lavender oil

1. Combine all ingredients in a blender, and blend until smooth.

2. Apply soak to dry hair, wrapping with plastic wrap. Keep treatment on hair for 30–60 minutes.

3. Rinse with warm water.

Hair or Nails Growth Serum

Strengthening, soothing, and stimulating with all-natural ingredients that protect the biological foundation of nails and hair, this versatile recipe can be used for nails or hair, leaving both strong and healthy, and ready for powerful growth!

INGREDIENTS | MAKES 2½ CUPS

¼ cup aloe vera gel

¼ cup vitamin E oil

2 cups brewed green tea, chilled

2–4 drops lavender oil

1. Combine all ingredients in a blender, and blend until thoroughly combined.

2. For nails, pour ½ cup solution into a shallow bowl and soak nails for 15–30 minutes daily.

3. For hair, apply ½–1 cup of solution to dry hair, cover with plastic wrap, and leave on hair for 30–60 minutes before rinsing with warm water.

CHAPTER 7

Aloe Vera and Weight

Ensuring your diet includes everything you need and none of what you don't can be challenging. Opting for salads, fruit, protein, healthy fats, and plenty of water are the nutritional keys that help achieve lasting weight loss, optimal muscle mass, and a healthy weight for years to come. Entwined in the mix of achieving and maintaining a healthy weight and body composition are not just food choices, but activity levels, lifestyle factors, and even mood. Aloe has shown to improve the rate of weight loss, and it's simple to see how: With myriad nutrients and phytochemicals that improve the functioning of your body's systems while focusing on the key factors that contribute to achieving lasting weight loss, aloe vera may just be the dietary addition you've been searching for.

Weight Loss and Maintenance

Every year, in the United States, Americans spend more than $20 billion on weight-loss products. From pills and potions to videos and diet clubs, the weight-loss industry's "empty promises for purchase" make big claims about products that provide results with little or no effort required, but usually fail to deliver.

The Dieting Cycle

For the more than 108 million dieters who make an average of four to five attempts at losing weight each year, the yo-yo lifestyle of roller-coaster dieting filled with ups and downs in hunger levels, weight gain and loss, and elation and depression are enough to make anyone feel like a failure.

These feelings only contribute to the cyclic process that landed most people in the weight-loss game to begin with: 1) overeating leads to weight gain, 2) weight gain leads to less energy and a reduced desire to work out, 3) lack of motivation to work out leads to more weight gain and a tendency to self-blame, 4) added weight and negative feelings lead to emotional eating with a higher tendency to overeat, returning to number 1, and the cycle begins again. But you can put a stop to the cycle and start a new path to the perfect weight for you.

A Natural Weight-Loss Aid

In order to be successful with weight loss or weight maintenance, you have to identify what your body needs, what changes you need to make, and how you can make improvements to your life naturally that will support your body as it transforms to a healthier state. As you go through the process of losing weight and maintaining that weight loss, you'll see how aloe vera can help improve your life, increase your results, and help you maintain a long-lasting level of health you never thought possible.

Aloe vera is not a magic pill or potion; it is an all-natural element that provides nutrients and phytochemicals that support your healthy lifestyle and improve your results by ensuring that your body's needs are being met. While it may sound "too good to be true," like the gimmicks that promise weight loss in a pill or a gadget, aloe vera differs in that it targets the body's overall health and improves the conditions of the body that contribute to a healthy weight effectively and naturally.

FACT

An astounding 95 percent of people who lose weight regain the lost weight within one year. Aloe vera provides nutrients and phytochemicals that can improve the functioning of the metabolic, hormonal, digestive, and thought processes that can contribute to the maintenance of healthy weight loss by helping your body readjust to its new, healthier weight.

Sadly, every day, millions of people work tirelessly to improve calorie burn and cut calories from their diet, spending hours at the gym or dieting on the latest fad diet. Few of those millions know what the contributing factors to weight loss and lasting weight maintenance are, and even fewer have organized their lifestyle to include those factors. These factors are simple and include only four areas of focus: energy, exercise, nutrition, and mood, each of which can be helped with the simplest addition of just 25 ml of aloe vera three times daily. Taken with your water, tea, or coffee, the naturally occurring elements of aloe vera can assist your body, its systems, and every one of its functions, helping to improve the four areas of focus essential for lasting weight loss and weight maintenance.

Body Composition: All Pounds Are Not Created Equally

There is no magic weight number that fits everyone, or even everyone of a certain size. People have different body compositions that contribute to the different body shapes and sizes that make us unique, and that variance in composition is what allows two people of the same size and shape to vary in weight by as much as 10–20 pounds but look almost exactly the same.

The difference in size is due to the body's composition, namely the ratio of muscle to fat. A pound of fat and a pound of muscle may weigh the same, but the difference in these two elements contributes to various effects in terms of your body's look, structure, and functioning. In the woman who exercises frequently and adheres to a clean diet free of processed foods, the higher proportion of heavier muscle mass contributes to her longer and leaner look that enables her to appear thinner than the other woman who, while weighing the same, has higher body fat content.

Those same pounds of fat and muscle also provide completely different benefits to the body and its functions. Muscle engages in a number of functions that require far more energy than fat; in the same time that it takes a pound of fat to burn 2 calories, a pound of muscle burns 6, all while the muscle is engaged in protein synthesis and countless other biochemical reactions that improve the functioning of the entire body. With the improved muscle mass composition comes higher fat-burning potential, too, helping your fat composition reduce throughout the process! Knowing the difference between muscle and fat, you can see why a body composition of more muscle and less fat is far more beneficial in the pursuit of healthier functioning and long-lasting weight loss.

ESSENTIAL

When the gut has a positive balance of microbe-combatting bacteria that beneficially combat serious digestive disorders, the surprising result can be better weight loss. With nutrients that support the natural digestive processes and ensure the proper absorption of essential nutrients, all while maintaining strong immunity against illness and disease, it is easier to lose weight and maintain weight loss.

Aloe vera can help immensely in the pursuit of improving your body's composition. Aloe vera not only contributes to the processes that help your body build muscle, but regular consumption of aloe can actually help your body maintain that muscle as you acquire it as well. By improving your body's ability to absorb the nutrients muscles require, improving the functioning of the circulatory system that provides the blood flow muscles need, and purging the blood of the lactic acid buildup that develops in muscles following exercise, aloe vera can be one of the most beneficial muscle-improving aspects of your daily routine.

Energy and Exercise

Without energy it is nearly impossible to achieve lasting weight loss. Food provides the calories that give your body the energy it needs to function, and those calories that are not used for activity get stored as fat. A sedentary lifestyle only adds more hurdles between you and your target weight, creating a larger obstacle to overcome as time progresses. Luckily, in terms of energy the adage "the more you use, the more you have" rings true. As your body works to perform bodily functions, tasks, and exercise, you expend energy. When your energy expenditure increases, your body reacts by using more fuel to prepare adequate energy for the next bout of work, expecting the increased energy output to happen again. Once this process is repeated enough, your body grows accustomed to the new procedure and automatically prepares itself time and time again. This means an improved calorie burn, increased energy levels, and a faster metabolism.

In order to use energy in the most beneficial way for achieving weight loss, you must exercise! Exercise can include a number of various activities, with the two most popular being cardiovascular activity and strength training.

Cardiovascular Training

Cardiovascular activities are those in which the body experiences an increase in heart rate for extended periods of time. Some examples of cardiovascular activities include walking, running, swimming, and biking. These activities challenge the body's muscles and result in a calorie burn during the actual activity, and for approximately 2–4 hours following the activity. Cardiovascular activity improves the functioning of the circulatory system and elicits positive responses from the brain in terms of serotonin and dopamine production.

FACT

By alternating exercise routines to focus on various aspects of the body's ability and functioning, you can improve your overall health exponentially. With a routine that alternates cardiovascular exercise, strength-training exercises, and flexibility training, the body and its systems are able to benefit from various challenges placed upon it when engaged in different activities.

Strength Training

When people hear "weight training," they often associate the phrase with large bodybuilders, but that connection could not be further from the truth. While specific programs using weights can produce large muscles, the goal of the average person's strength-training routine is simply to increase strength and improve muscle ability. With strength training, a routine that focuses on "low weight, high repetitions" (for long, lean muscles) or "high weight, low repetitions" (for bulky, large muscles) results in tiny tears in the muscle that the body must repair over the course of 24–48 hours, and it is over this entire period of time that calories are being burned and the metabolism experiences an increase.

How Aloe Vera Can Help

Aloe vera is not only able to supply the body with additional essential nutrients that contribute to the production of energy, but it is also able to improve the functioning of the cardiovascular system and multiple supporting systems that contribute to the healthy functioning of the body needed for energy output (exercise). With its store of B vitamins, aloe vera helps the body produce energy and improves the manufacturing and output of the hormones released during exercise that contribute to energy production and the "high" experienced during exercise.

Helping to improve the flow of the circulatory system, aloe also ensures that the delivery of essential energy-producing nutrients throughout the body remains efficient regardless of the activity in which the body is engaged. By providing the body with a variety of nutrients like B vitamins, vitamin C, iron, magnesium, anthraquinones, and antioxidants, aloe is able to support overall health before, during, and after the production and utilization of energy.

Metabolism

Your metabolism is the actual process your body uses to transform your consumed foods into energy. The energy produced through metabolism can be used for four areas of energy expenditure:

- The unseen functions like respiration, circulation, and digestion
- The body's process of digesting, absorbing, transporting, and storing nutrients after consumption of food
- Nonexercise physical activity (daily functions not intended to be exercise)
- Physical activity strenuous enough to be classified as "exercise"

QUESTION

What is nonexercise physical activity?
Whether you're cleaning your house, walking around your office, or grocery shopping, your body is engaged in physical activity. While this physical activity may not be considered as exercise, the motion and movement involved in the activity promotes calorie burn, muscle use, and physical demand on the body's functions.

BMR (Basal Metabolic Rate)

Your basal metabolic rate is the rate at which your body burns the calories it needs to maintain proper system functioning at rest, and this is where the majority of calorie burn takes place. Used to regulate the body's temperature, circulation, respiration, digestion, nerve impulses, etc., the BMR is a constant calorie-burning machine that helps your body stay alive. Determined by your sex, size, body composition, and age, the basal metabolic rate required to perform bodily functions and processes varies from person to person, but only varies slightly in terms of the percentage of daily caloric expenditure. On average, though, the BMR is responsible for between 60–75 percent of the calorie expenditure each and every day.

Thermic Effect

The thermic effect is the process associated with your body's response to a meal. In chewing, swallowing, digesting, processing, transporting, and storing, your body expends about 10 percent of its daily calories on the processes related to the thermic effect. As with the BMR, this caloric expenditure varies slightly among the population depending upon gender, size, etc., but that variance is limited and is nowhere near the variance of the area of thermogenesis.

Thermogenesis

Thermogenesis is defined as the process of an organism's generation of heat as a result of physical, physiological, and biological processes. In respect to the metabolism, there are two areas of thermogenesis that require calories: nonexercise activity thermogenesis and exercise activity thermogenesis.

NEAT (Nonexercise Activity Thermogenesis)

Beyond the BMR and the thermic effect, the body requires an additional percentage of calories to function physically in completing everyday tasks like walking, standing, bending, lifting, and even talking. Because these processes require a percentage of calories, the NEAT area is taken into consideration when calculating a metabolism because the variance among people in terms of the calories burned while working or at home can be significant depending upon the physical requirements of their day. While there may be a difference in caloric expenditure in this area, it is still somewhat comparable across populations and carries nowhere near the calorie-burning potential of EAT.

EAT (Exercise Activity Thermogenesis)

Exercise results in calorie burn, and the percentage of calories burned through physical activity contributes to the largest portion of disparity in the metabolism of people. While other factors of the metabolism could vary up to hundreds of calories at the most, this area of metabolism can have a variance of up to 2,000–5,000 calories between two people if one is extremely sedentary and the other extremely active.

The exercise activity thermogenesis area of the metabolism proves to be significant in contributing to overall weight loss and healthy weight maintenance, but all aspects of metabolic processes contribute to the overall calorie burn and need support to function properly. In contributing a number of supportive nutrients like the B vitamins and vitamin C, assorted minerals like iron and magnesium, and a number of amino acids, aloe vera can improve the daily calorie burn and improve weight loss and make sustaining that weight loss easier. By supporting the body's needs related to its everyday functions that contribute to the BMR, thermic effect, and thermogenesis, aloe vera has proven to be one of the most effective weight loss aids available.

Nutrition and Deficiencies

In order to function, your body needs various amounts of each of the macronutrients (carbohydrates, proteins, and fats) and micronutrients (vitamins and minerals). With clean sources of food providing your body with ample amounts of quality nutrition, these elements are taken in by the body and delivered to each system to perform a staggering number of functions.

Between the circulatory, muscular, lymphatic, digestive, nervous, and skeletal systems (plus many more) all running like efficient machines around the clock to contribute their own part to your overall health, it is imperative that the nutrients needed to promote and support your health and wellness are present.

One of the most notable areas of the body that shows the consumption of quality nutrition (or lack of it!) is your weight. In order to function properly, your body needs proteins, fats, carbohydrates, amino acids, and every single vitamin and mineral. With whole foods like fruit and vegetables, your body can use top-quality forms of nutrition to function not just properly, but optimally. When the body lacks a certain nutrient, or has chronic bouts of insufficient amounts of a nutrient, the issues can be widespread and affect a variety of functions, one being weight loss.

Because adequate nutrition plays such a critical role in weight loss and weight maintenance, aloe vera can improve the effectiveness of your diet and maximize your weight-loss potential. With ample amounts of vitamins and minerals that contribute to weight loss, as well as amino acids, enzymes, and sterols, aloe vera ensures your diet is not only supportive of weight loss, but also improves the body's absorption and utilization, improving overall health as well as weight-loss success!

Protein

With too little protein, your body suffers from fatigue and has a tendency to forage the body for protein sources, turning to muscle for the greatest source available for use in energy production. With ample amounts of protein in a diet, the body is able to produce energy, experience longer periods of fullness, and maintain muscle mass through a weight-loss program. Aloe vera supports the protein aspect of the diet by providing a number of essential amino acids required to produce and maintain muscle mass as well as the functions of those muscles.

FACT

Not only can protein help reduce cravings and increase feelings of fullness for longer durations, but this essential macronutrient has also shown to play a major role in weight loss long-term. Through improved metabolic functioning, diets higher in protein than carbohydrates and fats have shown to produce greater weight loss that continues for longer than diets with more comparative ratios of protein: carbs: fats.

Vitamin D

Because vitamin D–fortified products are everywhere on the market, this is the perfect place to point out that these products will never compare to acquiring D in its natural form through sun exposure. If a vitamin D deficiency occurs, the body reacts by experiencing a negative response to insulin, limiting the glucose transport to cells, signaling to the parathyroid hormone that calories should be stored as fat. This deficiency is also characterized by a reduction of the hormone leptin, which signals to the brain the feeling of fullness. Aloe vera helps in this area by protecting the skin from damaging UVA and UVB rays while being exposed to the sunlight that provides vitamin D.

Calcium

One of the little-known facts about calcium is that it can be found stored in fat cells, the GI tract, and the bloodstream. It is in every one of these areas that calcium acts to prevent excess weight gain and improve fat loss. In the fat cells, the more calcium that is available, the more fat is burned; in the GI tract, the more calcium that is available, the more it is able to bind to fat molecules and transport them out of the body via the liver rather than having them absorbed in the bloodstream. Aloe vera is very useful when it comes to calcium, as it aids in the absorption of the essential mineral.

ESSENTIAL

Don't forget about the power of positive thinking in your weight-loss plan. Aloe vera can improve the processes that contribute to positive thought. With healthy provisions of B vitamins, vitamin C, and vitamin E, the brain reacts positively with increased production of the "feel-good hormones," serotonin and dopamine, which improve the overall happiness factor and make you feel better about yourself and your weight-loss progress.

Iron

With enough iron in the blood, the body is able to do amazing things for weight loss. Conversely, when the iron supply is low, the cells and genes of the body react in ways that impede weight loss and actually contribute to weight gain. In times of iron deficiency, specific genes in the muscles and liver activate and signal the rest of the body that fat storage should increase; the result is not only a higher fat composition, but also abnormal blood sugar elevation. In terms of hormone activity, iron also is responsible for the communication with the T3 thyroid hormone that binds to cell membranes and communicates to nuclei about the rate of the metabolism. This prefaces more than eighty metabolic reactions that all require iron. If iron is in short supply, the reactions misfire and the result is a slow, ineffective metabolism. Aloe not only provides iron for the multiple processes involved in weight loss, but also the extraneous systems that contribute to those processes. Between ensuring proper hormone functioning, keeping the circulatory system free of issues and running properly, and improving the body's absorption of iron to be used throughout the body, aloe plays a major part in improving weight loss and maintaining that weight loss with better health to boot!

Recipes

Filling Fiber Green Smoothie

Fiber is essential for keeping your colon clear and ensuring the proper absorption of nutrients for the body's use. Fiber also makes you feel full longer.

INGREDIENTS | SERVES 2

¼ cup aloe vera juice

1 tablespoon ground flaxseed

1 cup chopped spinach

1 medium apple, peeled and cored

2 cups water, divided

1. Combine aloe, flaxseed, spinach, apple, and 1 cup water in a blender and blend until smooth.

2. Add remaining cup of water gradually and blend until desired consistency is achieved.

Colorful Corrector Smoothie

Aloe vera helps the body absorb vitamins A, B, C, and K, plus a number of essential minerals like zinc and potassium, to keep you strong and healthy.

INGREDIENTS | SERVES 2

¼ cup aloe vera juice

1 medium carrot, peeled and chopped

1 medium sweet potato, unpeeled

·1 cup chopped spinach

1 medium banana, peeled

2 cups water, divided

1. Combine aloe, carrot, sweet potato, spinach, banana, and 1 cup water in a blender and blend until smooth.

2. Add remaining cup of water gradually and blend until all ingredients are thoroughly combined.

Cherry Pick-Me-Up

With delicious ingredients like these, you'd never guess each sip is packed with powerful antioxidants that safeguard cells, improve metabolic functioning, and cleanse the blood. This smoothie is packed with natural caffeine—a delicious treat that can be enjoyed instead of coffee for a pick-me-up at any time of the day.

INGREDIENTS | SERVES 2

¼ cup aloe vera juice

2 cups brewed green tea, chilled

1 cup cherries, pitted and frozen

1 medium banana, peeled and frozen

Combine all ingredients in a blender. Blend until smooth.

Spicy Green Smoothie

The kick from natural cayenne not only helps improve the metabolism but can also help the body cleanse the blood of harmful levels of fatty deposits. Combine these benefits with the vitamins A, C, and K from the spinach and kale, and the natural antioxidants of tomatoes, green tea, and aloe, and you've got a perfect combination of health protection and health promotion in a single cup!

INGREDIENTS | SERVES 2

¼ cup aloe vera juice

2 cups brewed green tea, chilled

½ cup chopped spinach

½ cup chopped kale

½ large beefsteak tomato, chopped

½ teaspoon ground cayenne pepper

Combine all ingredients in a blender. Blend until smooth.

Spicy Metabolism Booster

Tasty, filling, and fueling the metabolism with essential protein and nutrients, this smoothie will provide energy, metabolic support, and filling fiber to help you achieve and maintain good health!

INGREDIENTS | SERVES 2

2 cups brewed green tea, chilled
¼ cup aloe vera juice
⅛ cup grated fresh gingerroot
1 teaspoon spirulina

Combine all ingredients in a blender. Blend until smooth.

CHAPTER 8

Digestive Issues

Digestive issues are some of the most commonly reported and prevalently treated health conditions in the world. Digestive issues can wreak havoc anywhere between the esophagus and the colon. With sufferers experiencing acute and mildly uncomfortable symptoms to consistent bouts of extremely painful or even debilitating attacks, digestive conditions can interfere with everyday life and adversely affect the quality of life. Regardless of the underlying cause, there are a number of preventative measures that can relieve the symptoms and even remedy the cause of digestive discomforts. One of the most effective treatments in the area of digestive issues is aloe vera. Contributing a number of essential elements that provide the body with nourishing nutrients, while supplying the digestive system with support, aloe vera can reduce the incidence of digestive issues and the severity of resulting symptoms. With serious conditions, it is always recommended to contact a medical professional before adding anything (including aloe vera) to your daily regimen. Serious conditions can be worsened by the attempt to self-treat without a medical professional's approval, so always consult your doctor before aloe vera applications are introduced.

Heartburn

The condition that most people refer to as heartburn is actually the symptom of a common condition called gastroesophageal reflux disease, or GERD. Heartburn is described as the hot burning sensation that rises up from the stomach or abdominal area into the esophagus beneath the chest or sternum area. In children, the symptoms of GERD can actually present themselves as dry coughs or trouble swallowing, and can be commonly misdiagnosed as asthma symptoms. While the experience of heartburn can be quite uncomfortable, the more serious concern is irreparable damage done to the esophagus by the consistent acid erosion when the acid rises from the stomach into the esophagus. This repetitive exposure to stomach acid can even result in esophageal cancers.

ALERT

While a number of heartburn relievers were once recommended for the treatment of heartburn commonly experienced during pregnancy, new recommendations warn pregnant women about the possible dangers of charcoal-containing heartburn relievers. If pregnant, always make sure you consult your physician before taking any new product.

The treatments for the symptoms resulting from GERD are intended to neutralize the acid levels of the stomach and are called proton pump inhibitors. Because the stomach acid that is present in the stomach is required for proper digestion and nutrition absorption processes, the use of these treatment methods can actually exacerbate the issue rather than remedy it. Instead of reducing the overall acid levels of the stomach, a more natural and effective treatment method has been found in using aloe vera.

By providing a number of naturally alkalizing properties, aloe vera can be used to decrease the severity and prevalence of heartburn by neutralizing the acid that produces heartburn. In addition to these pH-regulating properties that help regulate the "burning" acidity levels in the stomach, the anti-inflammatory anthraquinones that are unique to aloe vera help regulate the esophagus's muscle spasms, preventing the rising of acid into the esophagus and reducing the inflammation of the esophagus and digestive tract caused by previous or present heartburn. While helping to relieve the pain and discomfort of heartburn, aloe vera also provides properties that act as natural analgesics, or pain relievers, helping minimize the painful aftereffects of acid erosion. With a simple daily dose of 1–3 tablespoons, you can alleviate the pain of heartburn and begin the reparative process that provides future relief of the condition.

Constipation

A digestive condition that costs Americans $725 million annually, constipation is an uncomfortable and possibly serious condition that is characterized by minimal bowel movements or difficulty passing bowel movements. While the "normal" digestive processes vary greatly from person to person with some people reporting three bowel movements each day and others reporting only two to three bowel movements each week, constipation can be defined with the same varying degree of disparity.

The experience of constipation is most widely accepted as being more than 3 days of no bowel movements, straining with bowel movements, producing extremely hard stools that are difficult to pass, and "incomplete evacuation" of stools.

The most common contributing factors to constipation include a lack of water and fiber in the diet, medications, excessive dairy consumption, inadequate physical exercise, stress, or regular consumption of antacids. With a focus on improving these contributing factors, one can improve the regularity of bowel movements and reduce the incidence of constipation.

FACT

There is no question that raw aloe can produce a laxative effect. Even the simple handling of the cut leaf and its inner filet can produce a laxative effect within twenty-four hours. For constipation sufferers, this side effect can actually be a natural treatment option for chronic constipation.

Aloe vera has been proven to be an effective treatment method for constipation. The two unique properties of aloe vera, barbaloin and isobarbaloin, combine to produce the powerful compound commonly referred to as aloe vera latex. The aloe vera latex helps improve constipation by being processed in the large intestine and producing metabolites that induce bowel movements. In addition to the barbaloin and isobarbaloin, aloe vera also contains a compound named aloe emodin that inhibits the absorption of water in the digestive system and results in softer stools that are easier to form and pass.

With prolonged use of laxative medications, the digestive system can become dependent on the purgative effects of the medication, lessening the physical response required to evacuate the bowels naturally. While aloe's effects are similar to those of over-the-counter laxative medications, the results of aloe are naturally occurring and do not result in a possibility of dependence.

With a number of constipation aids, it is commonly reported that an abnormal loss of fluids and electrolytes can lead to dehydration. Because of the high water content of aloe vera (aloe is 99 percent water) and the high nutrient value that combines to create hydrating and electrolyte balancing benefits, aloe vera can provide constipation relief without harsh side effects, and it also has the added benefit of helping return regularity to bowel movements. The regular consumption of the recommended daily dose of 1–3 tablespoons of aloe vera can not only provide immediate relief, but also prevent future instances of constipation.

Stomach Ulcers

Stomach ulcers are also referred to as peptic ulcers because of the enzymatic stomach acid (pepsin) that contributes to the formation and pain resulting from ulcers. More than 25 million Americans will experience the discomfort of an ulcer at some point in their lives. This staggering percentage of the population will spend millions of dollars in treatment methods to cure the condition, ranging from antacids and medications to endoscopy procedures and even hospitalizations if the condition is not cared for properly.

Surprisingly, one of the contributing factors to ulcers is the use of NSAID (nonsteroidal anti-inflammatory drugs) pain relievers like ibuprofen. Unknowingly, many people suffering from ulcerative conditions and symptoms turn to NSAID pain relievers for relief, which actually worsen the condition rather than improving it. The most likely contributing factors to peptic ulcers are lifestyle-related issues such as stress, smoking, alcohol consumption, and a diet of high-fat or highly acidic foods, but the underlying issue that actually causes an ulcer is the bacteria *H. pylori.*

Ulcers are the result of damage to the protective layer of the mucus that lines the digestive system from the esophagus through the intestine. When the wearing down of this protective layer occurs, open sores (ulcers) result. Because this bacteria is able to thrive in the digestive system, the condition of an ulcer can worsen over time if not treated. Without a proper diagnosis through an endoscopy to determine the actual presence of an ulcer, it can be hard to actually identify the causes of the upset stomach, heartburn, vomiting, diarrhea, etc., because the symptoms may come and go, rather than remaining chronic indications of a serious issue. The most common treatment for an ulcer is a combination of an antibiotic to kill the bacterial infection and a diet regimen that refrains from fatty or acidic foods, or those high in sugar and starch (which can feed a bacteria and further exacerbate the ulcer being treated).

FACT

Sometimes foods and genetics aren't the only factors that contribute to the development or progression of ulcers. Many people who suffer from ulcers can find relief from the chronic condition by engaging in stress-reducing activities. By meditating, engaging in exercise, journaling, and relaxing, an ulcer sufferer may be able to find natural relief.

As opposed to the most accepted antibiotic in the treatment of ulcers that kills all bacteria and microbes throughout the body, aloe vera has been shown to be a safe and healthy alternative in treating ulcers. Aloe vera provides the body with naturally occurring phytochemicals that act to fight harmful microbes, bacteria, viruses, and fungi, while preserving the helpful bacteria, microbes, and fungi that can safeguard your health. The loss of essential microbes, bacteria, and fungi can lead to candida overgrowth in the digestive system and a reduced immunity, which can cause further health complications.

To further protect the immune system and relieve the pain associated with ulcers, aloe vera provides naturally occurring antioxidants and anthraquinones that combine to provide protection against infection, inflammation, and even pain. With these compounds acting to minimize the physical reaction to an ulcer while preventing pain receptors from communicating pain experiences, aloe vera can reduce the chances of further infection and harmful changes while also helping to relieve pain naturally. Aloe also contains a number of helpful enzymes and phyto-chemicals that contribute to the healing process; just as aloe has been shown to be effective in the treatment of skin conditions, the same prop-erties responsible for faster healing times externally can be used for improved healing internally. The recommended daily dose of just 1–3 tablespoons of aloe vera has been shown to reduce the pain of ulcers, help speed the healing process, and reduce the chances of developing ulcers in the future.

Inflammatory Bowel Disease (IBD)

Inflammatory bowel disease is comprised of two different diseases: Crohn's disease and ulcerative colitis. While having very similar signs and symp-toms, these two diseases differ in a number of areas that are great enough to warrant a distinction.

Crohn's Disease

Crohn's disease is characterized by chronic inflammation of the gastrointestinal tract. While this disease can be widespread throughout the GI tract, it has a tendency to affect the end of the bowel predominately. The inflammation associated with Crohn's disease occurs as a result of the good bacteria in the gastrointestinal areas being misidentified as foreign invaders. Wrongly attacking these helpful bacteria, cells travel out of the bloodstream and move into the gastrointestinal area to attack, which leads to inflammation. With this disease, the inflammation never subsides and becomes a chronic condition that leads to ulceration within the lining of the gastrointestinal tract and thickening of the intestinal wall.

The symptoms of this disease range from abdominal pain and cramping to bloody stools that can be loose and persistent. Compounding the difficulty of dealing with this painful disease is the fact that there is no known cause or cure. While there may be a genetic predisposition for the disease, there is no known evidence supporting the direct link among family members.

Ulcerative Colitis

Similar to Crohn's disease, ulcerative colitis also has no known cause or cure. The symptoms of ulcerative colitis are also similar to Crohn's in that the discomfort can range from minor or severe abdominal cramping to bloody stools that can lead to further complications such as anal fissures and tears.

Ulcerative colitis differs from Crohn's disease in that the reaction that leads to the inflammation is spiked by food entering the gastrointestinal tract; once food enters the digestive tract, the body perceives it as a threat and sends white blood cells to attack. The inflammation that results from this attack leads to ulcers throughout the colon that further exacerbate the inflammation by leaking pus and mucous. The inflammation and ulcers occur only in the colon and are specific to the internal lining (unlike Crohn's, which attacks every layer of the wall).

While Crohn's can leave patches of the gastrointestinal tract unharmed, ulcerative colitis damages the entire lining of the colon, leaving the entire area inflamed and affected by the pus and mucous it exudes from the ulcers. While there is no known cure for this disease, the flare-ups that lead to the physical symptoms can have long periods of remission between in which no symptoms are experienced.

Aloe for IBD

With no known causes or cures for inflammatory bowel disease, the treatment methods can yield minimal results and rarely help reduce the incidence of symptoms, minimize future flare-ups, or reverse damage caused by the chronic inflammation. In utilizing aloe vera and its naturally occurring properties, sufferers can safely and effectively minimize contributing factors while also treating both the symptoms and the damage.

With its provision of anthraquinones acting as powerful anti-inflammatory agents, aloe is able to minimize the inflammation that results in the physical symptoms of IBD. With ample amounts of vitamins and minerals that can correct possible deficiencies that result from inadequate absorption during digestion, aloe may also be able to minimize future flare-ups.

For ulcers and irritations that are commonly seen in IBD patients, aloe vera can help prevent the growth of harmful bacteria and microbes, while encouraging the growth of beneficial bacteria that can assist in the reparation and prevention of ulcers. In addition, aloe vera's amino acids and enzymes can contribute to the improvement of nerve cell health throughout the body, allowing for improved regulation of response within the areas of the GI tract affected by IBD as well as in the brain, helping improve the physical response to the nerve messages from within the GI tract. With a daily dose of 1–3 tablespoons of aloe vera, one can improve the health of the digestive system, prevent pain associated with IBD, and minimize the chances of future IBD flare-ups.

Irritable Bowel Syndrome (IBS)

Irritable bowel syndrome (IBS) may sound very similar to inflammatory bowel disease (IBD) but is different in that IBS consists of a group of temporary symptoms rather than the persistent, lifelong inflammation of IBD that classifies it as a chronic disease. IBS is referred to as a "functional gastrointestinal disorder" by the International Foundation for Gastrointestinal Disorders because the syndrome is a direct result of an error in functioning within the digestive system.

The symptoms of IBS can range from bloating and abdominal pain that subside after a bowel movement to changes in bowel movement consistency and diarrhea or constipation. Diet, stress, menstrual periods, changes in routine, etc., have long been thought to contribute to the incidence of IBS and its symptoms, but further examination and study has determined a higher prevalence of IBS with brain-gut signal dysfunction and overly sensitive nerve endings in the GI tract.

Medical professionals theorize that when the communication between the gut and the brain is malfunctioning, the result can be an overly active GI tract; accurately termed "irritable" bowel syndrome, IBS may also be a result of easily irritated nerve endings in the GI tract that react to ordinary stimuli like food and ever-present GI bacteria with exaggerated responses.

Aloe can be very helpful in treating IBS and its symptoms with its natural provision of alkalizing elements that regulate pH and minimize acidity levels that could aggravate digestion and lead to IBS symptoms. With its healthy doses of amino acids and enzymes, aloe vera can also improve IBS by providing the building blocks necessary for proper protein synthesis and usage, helping reduce digestive issues and relieve stomach pain.

Aloe vera's anthraquinones can minimize the discomfort of IBS by preventing the formation of uncomfortable inflammatory conditions and minimizing the pain that can result. With its antiseptic properties aloe vera is able to cleanse the GI tract and produce laxative effects that keep the GI tract clean and free of possible irritants that could contribute to the development of symptoms.

Most importantly, aloe vera is able to provide healthy antioxidants and essential vitamins, minerals, and phytochemicals that improve and safeguard the connections and communications between the GI tract and the brain, helping reduce the incidence of improper functioning of the nerves within the GI tract and the improper stimulation by the brain that elicits the exaggerated response from the gut. With the numerous benefits of aloe vera on the digestive tract, one can minimize IBS flare-ups and associated symptoms with a simple daily dose of just 1–3 tablespoons of aloe vera.

Diverticulitis

Diverticulitis is a bowel disease that affects at least half of the population over the age of sixty at some point in their lives. Throughout the large intestine of a person with diverticulitis there are small areas of inflammation that create bulging sacs that act as pouches. In a normal digestive tract, feces is able to move through and be passed without incident, but in a person with diverticulitis bits of feces are trapped and blocked by the bulging pouches. These bits of excrement remain caught in the diverticula and can breed bacteria, leading to infection and inflammation. Characterized by a sudden onset of severe symptoms that include abdominal pain, fever, chills, nausea, and vomiting, diverticulitis is diagnosed with colonoscopy and possibly a CT scan. One of the most widely accepted natural treatments for diverticulitis is a combination of aloe vera and a liquid diet that progresses to a high-fiber diet.

In treating diverticulitis, aloe vera can provide a number of helpful properties that act to prevent the inflammation from occurring, improve digestion, remove remaining bits of food, and return the wall of the digestive system to a healthy state. With a number of phytochemicals that act as anti-inflammatory compounds, aloe vera can not only help minimize the inflammation that results from diverticulitis, but can also help in preventing flare-ups of inflammation that create the bulging sacs characterized by the disease. The anthraquinones in aloe vera also act as an effective treatment for inflammation as well as an effective prevention.

Aloe vera has long been known as an effective method of detoxing the digestive system and improving digestion by initiating the release of increased water in the digestive system; this benefit improves the condition of diverticulitis by literally flushing the bits of left-behind feces that cause irritation and inflammation. Through its ability to fight bacteria and viruses while maintaining a healthy balance of beneficial bacteria and flora in the gut, aloe is able to fend off the infection that precipitates the severe symptoms of diverticulitis while also providing pain-relieving compounds that can minimize the discomfort of the inflammation and resulting symptoms naturally! A daily dose of 1–3 tablespoons of aloe vera has been shown to provide relief from a number of digestive issues, including diverticulitis. Through the daily consumption of aloe vera, diverticulitis sufferers not only experience less frequent flare-ups, but also experience minimal symptoms associated with the condition when flare-ups do occur.

Gallstones

The painful experience of passing a gallstone is one that millions of Americans endure every year. With gallstones ranging in size from a grain of sand to larger than a golf ball, there's no wonder that one of the most common surgeries in the United States is gallbladder removal.

Gallstones form as a result of excess cholesterol in the bile. Bile is the necessary fluid comprised of cholesterol, bilirubin, and bile salts produced by the liver to aid in the digestion of food. Though the bile is produced by the liver, it is stored in the gallbladder to be secreted in the small intestine during digestion. When there is an excess of cholesterol in the gallbladder, small gallstones form that can quickly increase in number and size, resulting in pain in the abdomen and back, nausea, and vomiting. Obesity, diabetes, high estrogen levels, and cholesterol-reducing medications have been identified as the main culprits in contributing to the excessive levels of cholesterol that form gallstones.

Providing powerful phytochemicals and nutrients that directly affect the main precursors of gallstone development, aloe vera has been used as an effective method for prevention as well as treatment. Aloe vera provides unique plant sterols that reduce LDL (bad) cholesterol levels, improve HDL (good) cholesterol levels, and reduce the levels of triglycerides and total lipid levels. With these improvements, the issue of excess cholesterol is minimized and the incidence of gallstone formation is reduced dramatically. Further supporting the body's defenses against gallstones is aloe's ability to improve the hormone balance of the body, minimizing the excessive estrogen risk factor among men and women.

ALERT

The connection between diet and gallstones is serious enough to warrant attention. If you suffer from gallstones, you should consume a diet of high-fiber foods such as fruits and vegetables, beans, and nuts, and drink plenty of fluids (at least 2 liters per day). Avoid processed, high-fat foods, and minimize foods such as pastas and grains.

With the added benefits of healthier digestion and improved overall system functioning, aloe vera can not only minimize the risk factors and incidence of gallstones, but also improve your overall health! To minimize the development and symptoms related to gallstones, the recommended daily consumption of 1–3 tablespoons of aloe vera has shown to be extremely effective.

Recipes

Spicy Stomach Soother

While these ingredients may seem unorthodox, each contributes amazing benefits to the digestive system. Ginger calms the stomach, green tea provides antioxidants, and apple cider vinegar combats bacteria, viruses, and microbes. This stomach-soothing combo is not only beneficial, but delicious too!

INGREDIENTS | SERVES 2

2 cups brewed green tea, chilled

⅛ cup grated fresh gingerroot

1 tablespoon organic, unfiltered, and unpasteurized apple cider vinegar

4 ounces aloe vera juice

Combine all ingredients in a blender. Blend until smooth.

Apple-Beet Treat

Fiber-filled, antioxidant-rich, and containing tons of vitamins and minerals, this smoothie provides sweet relief from any kind of stomach discomfort!

INGREDIENTS | SERVES 2

¼ cup aloe vera juice

2 cups water

2 medium apples, peeled and cored

1 cup beet greens

2 medium roasted beets, cooled, peeled, and chopped

Combine all ingredients in a blender. Blend until smooth.

Sweet Protein Smoothie

Protein is an absolutely essential element that must be included in every meal and snack to maintain proper functioning of all the body's systems. Smoothies help you get your protein in easily.

INGREDIENTS | SERVES 2

¼ cup aloe vera juice

1 cup unsweetened vanilla almond milk

1 cup vanilla Greek yogurt

1 medium banana, peeled and frozen

⅛ cup ground flaxseed

Combine all ingredients in a blender. Blend until smooth.

Sweet Potato Pie Smoothie

The complex carbohydrates, fiber, and naturally occurring sugars of sweet potatoes star in this delicious diet-improving smoothie. Try sipping this smoothie when you crave something sweet, and you'll feel full and satisfied.

INGREDIENTS | SERVES 2

2 cups unsweetened almond milk

¼ cup aloe vera juice

1 medium sweet potato, cooked and peeled

1 teaspoon ground cinnamon

1 teaspoon ground cloves

½ cup ice

Combine all ingredients in a blender. Blend until smooth.

Hello, Hydration!

In addition to a daily 64 ounces of water, consider smoothies like this one that can add essential electrolytes and hydrating nutrients for longer-lasting hydration that has added benefits of nutrition!

INGREDIENTS | SERVES 2

¼ cup aloe vera juice

2 cups water

2 medium cucumbers, peeled and chopped

3 medium kiwifruit, peeled and chopped

Combine all ingredients in a blender. Blend until smooth.

CHAPTER 9

Chronic Diseases

Heart disease, stroke, cancer, diabetes, and obesity are the most common chronic diseases in the United States today. With a staggering 117 million Americans currently diagnosed with at least one of these conditions, more and more attention is being focused on methods of prevention. With a multitude of powerful health-improving compounds, supported by a long history of success in the treatment and prevention of serious illnesses, aloe vera may be able to help the chronic disease crisis and improve the health and lives of millions of people now and for years to come.

Heart Disease

The leading cause of death around the world is cardiovascular disease, with an average of 17.3 million people dying of heart disease every year. Researchers around the globe have spent decades trying to determine the exact cause of the diseases that comprise heart disease as a whole. While the entire cardiovascular system is affected by the onset of cardiovascular disease, six types of heart disease have been identified with each affecting a different area of the cardiovascular system:

- **Coronary heart disease**, a disease of the blood vessels that supply the heart muscle, is the most prevalent of all cardiovascular diseases.
- **Cerebrovascular disease** is a disease of the blood vessels that supply the brain.
- **Peripheral arterial disease** affects the blood vessels that supply the arms and legs.
- **Rheumatic fever** is caused by the streptococcal virus and causes damage to the heart's muscles and valves.
- **Congenital heart defects** are malformations of the heart structure that occur during development prior to birth.
- **Deep vein thrombosis** refers to blood clots in leg veins that dislodge and move to the heart, lungs, or brain, creating a pulmonary embolism.

In an effort to reduce the number of annual deaths that result from cardiovascular disease, the World Health Organization has identified prevention as the best defense against cardiovascular disease. Twenty percent of cardiovascular disease cases result from genetics, which means that 80 percent of the cases are a result of lifestyle choices. Behavioral factors that contribute to the development of heart disease include a poor diet, physical inactivity, smoking, and alcohol abuse.

Diet plays a crucial role in the development of cardiovascular disease by creating physical precursors to the disease's development. Creating a buildup of fatty deposits on the walls of blood vessels throughout the body, the diet and resulting conditions from a long history of poor dietary choices have shown to aggravate the specific areas of the cardiovascular system most affected by the disease by producing these fatty deposits and encouraging their growth for extended periods of time.

High blood pressure, hypertension, high blood lipids, diabetes, and obesity have all been identified as predisposing factors to cardiovascular disease. With a number of negative impacts to one's overall health, these conditions contribute to an unhealthy disruption in the body's natural balance of sugars, fats, and cholesterol; with these three components of the blood in high concentration, the blood vessel walls with thicker fat (or plaque) deposits inhibit the proper flow of the circulatory system and contribute to the rising risk of cardiovascular disease.

Aloe Can Help

With an impressive number of essential nutrients and powerful phytochemicals, aloe vera is able to improve the body's overall health, better the body's synergistic system functioning, and cleanse the blood, all helping to reduce the incidence of cardiovascular disease. Since diabetes and obesity play major roles in the development of cardiovascular disease, it is essential for anyone who has a lifestyle conducive to these conditions to make a serious effort to minimize the factors that contribute to their condition, and also to take the steps necessary to reverse the condition. In both of these areas, aloe vera can help immensely.

Aloe vera provides the dietary nutrients that help the body maintain proper system functioning, thereby helping the obese or diabetic patient minimize the disruptions of these systems. For example, aloe's vitamins A, C, and E can help minimize the oxidative stress placed on the body as a result of the conditions while also improving the immunity. Aloe's B vitamins and vitamin K combine to promote overall health and wellness by maintaining productive nerve cells and optimal communication between those nerves and the brain.

All these vitamins also support healthy lifestyle choices by improving energy levels (supporting activity), minimizing cravings for unhealthy foods, improving the absorption of essential nutrients, and optimizing the body's ability to eliminate fat and create muscle, all factors that contribute to the body's return to optimal health. With essential minerals like calcium, iron, and magnesium, aloe also supports the body's main components like muscle, blood, tissue, and bone. Without the health of these main structural components, disease and low energy levels can contribute to unhealthy lifestyle choices like inactivity while also making the body susceptible to a cascade of illnesses that can further aggravate conditions that contribute to cardiovascular disease.

ALERT

Obesity is one of the most common risk factors of chronic diseases. Not only can the condition complicate a healthy lifestyle by posing limitations on activities that would otherwise improve health, the excess weight and effort required to carry it can place unnecessary pressure on the body's organs.

The main provisions of aloe vera that foster improved cardiovascular health are found in the phytochemicals specific to aloe that act as cholesterol-improving, blood-cleansing agents. With the effects of aloe having been studied and proven to show improvements in the serum cholesterol levels, triglyceride levels, and total lipid levels of the blood (all being the identified precursors for cardiovascular disease), you can see how aloe vera can help improve the health of an at-risk patient, reducing the chances of developing cardiovascular disease dramatically.

With a regular and consistent daily dose of 1–3 tablespoons of aloe vera, a sufficient amount of the vitamins, minerals, antioxidants, and phytochemicals associated with reducing the risk for the development of heart disease can be provided throughout the body.

Stroke

Like a heart attack that results from a reduced flow of blood and oxygen to the heart, a stroke is a "brain attack" that results from a decrease in the flow of blood and oxygen to the brain. In the United States, there is an estimated one stroke every 40 seconds, and one stroke-induced death every 4 minutes. Every year, there are approximately 795,000 strokes, with women suffering from 55,000 more strokes than men, annually. Because strokes are the result of a mishap in the cardiovascular system, this condition is commonly grouped with those resulting from cardiovascular disease.

ESSENTIAL

Whether you choose to add aloe vera to your water, coffee, or tea, or pour it over your favorite salads and sides, this natural wonder can be seamlessly implemented into your day. Tasting similar to water, this tasteless, odorless addition can go unnoticed, but it provides plenty of benefits to every area of your life!

Types of Strokes

Strokes are divided into two subcategories (ischemic and hemorrhagic) depending upon the cause of the stroke. Ischemic strokes make up a majority of all strokes experienced, with an estimated 87 percent of all strokes being due to this condition. In an ischemic stroke, arteries are blocked by blood clots, plaque buildup, or fatty deposits, drastically reducing the blood and oxygen flow to the brain, or cutting off the brain's supply completely. A hemorrhagic stroke occurs when a blood vessel in the brain bursts or breaks, causing bleeding in the brain. Both of these strokes, while different, are equally deadly and can be prevented with the same measures.

Contributing Factors

The National Stroke Association has outlined a number of factors that can directly and indirectly contribute to the experience of a stroke. An unhealthy diet, inactivity, high blood pressure, high cholesterol, existing heart disease, and diabetes all contribute to the prevalence of strokes. An improved diet including maximum nutrients, an increased awareness of one's state of health, and the proven benefits of aloe vera can only improve the chances of avoiding the possibility of stroke. A simple addition of 1–3 tablespoons of aloe vera to your daily routine can drastically improve the functioning of the brain and the body, helping to minimize the chances of developing the risk factors connected with strokes.

ALERT

The most commonly reported symptom of a stroke stems from the actual malfunctioning of the brain; many stroke sufferers report that their first indication that something was wrong was either the inability to understand or communicate, or a sudden feeling of numbness or paralysis on the face or one side of the body.

Cancer

Cancer is defined as the uncontrollable growth of abnormal cells in the body. Also called malignant cells, these cancerous changes at a cellular level can occur in any type of tissue throughout the body. Striking every area from the skin to the bones, the brain to the heart, and every organ throughout the body, cancerous cells can develop and spread rapidly, even metastasizing from one organ or area to another in rapid succession. Because many cancers are asymptomatic (showing no signs or symptoms that cancer is developing), many cancer sufferers are unaware that they have cancer until advanced stages are reached. The early diagnosis of cancer is the most beneficial aspect of cancer treatment.

The causes of cancer can be as numerous as the types of cancers. A staggering number of elements to which people have been exposed for generations have now been deemed unsafe cancer causers that not only contribute to the cancerous changes at the cellular level, but also exacerbate the speed of cancer growth and its spread. Exposure to sunlight and toxins such as cigarette smoke and alcohol have been attributed to the growth of cancer, while pre-existing conditions like obesity and diabetes have also been named as possible contributing factors in the development of the disease. Because each and every risk associated with the development of cancers (aside from the genetic predisposition) is based on healthy or unhealthy lifestyle choices, a growing number of physicians have turned their focus to promoting the "prevention is the best medicine" tactic in reducing the prevalence of cancer.

ESSENTIAL

Many people claim to have found the cure for cancer. While studies are ongoing, the September 2012 issue of *BioMedicine* featured a study by Shu-Chun Hsu that reported the effectiveness of emodin (an aloe anthraquinone) in the arresting of cancer tumor cells' growth. For more information on this study, please see the citation in the appendix.

The Cancer Treatment Debate

In terms of treatment, there is a wide variance of opinion. Some medical professionals recommend rigorous methods of cancer-killing drugs and others promote nutrition and lifestyle changes. The best-known cancer treatments, chemotherapy and radiation, have long been considered the best treatment options for curing cancer. However, they have become the source of heated debates recently because these methods identify and kill not only cancerous cells, but kill healthy cells as well. The maintenance of healthy cells is absolutely critical in the prevention, treatment, and recovery processes related to cancer. Without healthy cells, the body becomes less resistant to disease, infection, and abnormal changes, creating a "perfect storm" scenario that can result in a return of cancer, or worse.

Those promoting the nutritional treatment methods belong to the branch of medicine known as alternative medicine. With a number of studies that attribute specific health benefits to the use of vitamins and minerals, as well as phytochemicals, these alternative medicine proponents promote the use of nutrition for the prevention and treatment of cancer. With the applications of these natural nutrients to the body, some believe that the nutrients and antioxidants provided by aloe vera can provide benefits that help cancerous cells diminish in size and number, healthy cells increase in number, and improve the overall functioning of the immune system (helping maintain strong immunity and overall quality health while undergoing treatment). Alternative medical practitioners feel that because the cancerous cells are minimized and destroyed while healthy cells and systems benefit from improved health, the natural methods of administering nutrients as cancer treatment should be given more attention.

How Aloe Can Help During Treatment

With its staggering provision of natural antioxidants, aloe vera's vitamins A, C, and E, and naturally occurring sterols and enzymes, act to directly improve the health of cells; this antioxidant support is the premise behind the assumption sparking scientific studies delving into the possibility that aloe vera may be an effective treatment for cancer by minimizing cancerous changes and improving the number of healthy cells and effectiveness of white blood cells. Aloe's powerful antiseptic agents support the work of the antioxidants by minimizing the health-deteriorating elements within the blood and tissues, improving overall health while minimizing the workload of reparative cells that are needed at the site of cancerous changes. Maintaining an effective immune system is absolutely crucial while the body's defenses are low due to the effects of cancerous changes, and aloe vera's ability to act as an antibacterial, antiviral, antifungal, and antimicrobial agent can help safeguard the body from harmful irritants, minimizing the workload on the immune system and allowing the immune system to fully focus on the cancerous areas in need. Lastly, the vitamins, amino acids, and enzymes of aloe vera combine to help the cancer-stricken patient maintain energy levels, proper hormone balance, and efficient nutrient processing that all combine to help the entire body function optimally.

The use of aloe vera may also be an effective treatment for side effects resulting from the chemotherapy drugs and radiation treatment used to kill cancerous cells, with its proven ability to treat radiation burns. In addition aloe is effective in repairing digestive issues and symptoms, which may benefit cancer patients with some of the other debilitating side effects that stem from cancer treatments.

Diabetes

Diabetes is a metabolic disease in which the body is not able to produce enough insulin, resulting in high levels of glucose in the blood. While this condition's definition sounds simplistic, the disease can be catastrophic, costing one American life every three minutes. The World Health Organization has determined that more than 382 million people, worldwide, suffer from diabetes, and the number of Americans dealing with the disease has increased by 40 percent to 29 million in just ten years. Killing more than AIDS and breast cancer combined, the deaths attributed to diabetes represent a fraction of the catastrophic results that are caused by the disease; as the leading cause of amputations (not sustained by injury), blindness, kidney failure, heart failure, and stroke, diabetes not only claims lives, but also slowly deteriorates the lives of diabetes patients. With an expected doubling of diabetes patients by the year 2030, diabetes has become a major concern, not only for today, but for the future of the entire world's population as well.

Diabetes is a disease that results from a consistently affected level of blood sugar, or glucose, in the bloodstream resulting from the body's inability to properly process glucose. When you eat, your body turns food into glucose, a form of sugar that is used to generate energy within the cells. The glucose signals a response from the pancreas to release insulin. The three different types of diabetes are type 1, type 2, and gestational.

Type 1 Diabetes

Also referred to as insulin-dependent diabetes, type 1 diabetes is an autoimmune disorder in which the body perceives the pancreatic cells as foreign invaders and attacks them, thereby inhibiting the body's production of insulin and the processing of glucose. The destroyed pancreatic cells, called islets, are responsible for sensing glucose and producing a necessary amount of insulin. When the insulin is supposed to be released into the bloodstream, the destroyed pancreatic cells don't produce enough insulin or produce no insulin at all. The disrupted process prevents the body's cells from collecting the glucose for energy production because the insulin required for the process is not available. The failure of the cells to intake the glucose produces a catastrophic domino effect; when the cells don't receive glucose, they not only starve, but also leave the unprocessed glucose in the bloodstream, resulting in high blood glucose or high blood sugar levels.

Type 2 Diabetes

Type 2 diabetes is also referred to as insulin resistant. This type of diabetes normally strikes people as they age, warranting the alternative term *adult onset diabetes*, though more and more children and adolescents are developing this form of diabetes. With type 2 diabetes, the insulin that is produced is no longer enough for the glucose processing. This occurs due to muscle, liver, and fat cells no longer functioning optimally, failing to use the insulin for glucose delivery. The pancreas provides more insulin to compensate initially, but can't keep up with the demands for insulin and eventually needs assistance through medication or insulin injections.

Gestational Diabetes

Gestational diabetes is the type of diabetes that develops during pregnancy as a result of specific hormones being produced during the pregnancy that create insulin resistance. Normally subsiding following the delivery of the baby, gestational diabetes can lead to pregnancy complications and is considered a precursor for the development of type 2 diabetes later in life.

How Aloe Can Help

With the remarkable number of vitamins and minerals contained within it, aloe vera can help reduce the incidence of diabetes and its symptoms. The most effective aspect of aloe is due to its powerful phytochemicals. Two main concerns related to diabetes are the components of the blood that are adversely affected by the excess blood glucose and the inability to heal properly following an injury. The most widely accepted daily dose for ingested aloe is 1–3 tablespoons; through regular consumption of ⅓ of the daily dose, three times daily, a diabetic may be able to return blood sugar levels to normal and experience more frequent regularly stabilized numbers throughout the day. Topically, aloe vera can be applied to a diabetic's wound as often as necessary, in an amount that is sufficient to cover the wound in its entirety. Because of its effectiveness in reducing blood sugar, aloe vera should never be consumed while taking diabetic medication without first addressing the implementation of aloe vera with your physician.

Aloe vera is not only able to help improve healing time with ingested gel and topical applications at the site of an injury, but can also help improve the dangerous levels of glucose, cholesterol, lipids, and triglycerides that result from improper functioning of the pancreas and related cells. With anti-inflammatory, antioxidant, and blood-sugar-regulating properties, the aloe plant is able to provide helpful aloe-specific enzymes and naturally occurring compounds like plant sterols that help naturally reduce levels of bad cholesterol (LDL), improve levels of good cholesterol (HDL), regulate blood sugar levels, and reduce the lipids and triglycerides of the blood.

Obesity

In 2010, the Centers for Disease Control and Prevention released a report with a shocking statistic: more than ⅓ of the American adult population was obese, and a startling 20 percent of children ages two through nineteen were obese. Defined as an unhealthy accumulation of excessive body fat, obesity is not just an aesthetic condition that poses limitations, but a true disease that can lead to more serious conditions. With the number of obese individuals growing annually, and more and more children becoming obese, the need for awareness about the contributing factors and possible resulting conditions is apparent now more than ever. Having determined that the expenses of obesity-related healthcare costs have reached $190.2 million, or a whopping 21 percent of all healthcare spending in America, the World Health Organization (WHO) and the Centers for Disease Control and Prevention (CDC) have included obesity in the their lists of chronic diseases plaguing America, and the world as a whole.

Obesity is not a disease one contracts and develops overnight. After years of lifestyle choices that contribute to the development of excess body fat, obesity takes hold of the entire body. With poor dietary choices, a sedentary lifestyle, erratic sleep patterns, extensive use of medications, and smoking and alcohol consumption all playing a part in the development of body fat, obesity is the result of a deadly combination of lifestyle choices and habits. The most widely accepted diagnosis of obesity is the calculation of the body mass index (BMI), determining if a patient is more than 20 percent over the weight considered "normal" for his height.

Body Mass Index (BMI)

The most widely accepted calculation used to determine one's weight classification is the body mass index (BMI), which is calculated by dividing one's weight in kilograms by one's height in meters squared. With the resulting calculation, a person can determine where she falls in terms of predetermined classes that range from underweight to extremely obese.

For example, a person weighing 120 pounds who is 5'6" tall would use the following calculation to find her BMI:

1. Convert pounds to kilograms: $120 \times .453 = 54.43$
2. Convert inches to meters: 5'6" (66") $\times .0254 = 1.68$
3. Square the resulting metric conversion: $1.68^2 = 2.82$
4. Divide weight in kg by the height in meters squared: $54.43/2.82 = 19.3$

This resulting calculation of 19.3 would then be used in determining the class of that weight range, which includes all BMI calculations from 18.5 through 40:

- Underweight: less than 18.5
- Normal: 18.5–24.9
- Overweight: 25–29.9
- Obese (class I): 30–34.9
- Obese (class II): 35–39.9
- Extremely obese (class III): 40 and higher

The Effects of Obesity

Affecting the body's development, functioning, and systems, obesity wreaks havoc on the body by reducing the proficiency of the body's normal processes and contributing to the development of serious illnesses and diseases. As a result of obesity, a number of serious conditions can develop, all of which are further exacerbated by the excessive weight of the individual.

The health conditions that are directly related to excessive weight are high levels of bad cholesterol (LDL), low levels of good cholesterol (HDL), high blood pressure, heart disease, metabolic syndrome, stroke, cancer, respiratory diseases, arthritis, inflammation, and even skin conditions. With the onset of these resulting conditions, obesity not only limits one's abilities and adversely affects quality of life, but it also creates a perfect storm of symptoms and conditions that can lead to death.

How Aloe Can Help

Knowing the numerous benefits that aloe can have on the blood, brain, organs, and overall system functioning of the body, it's no surprise that aloe can help reduce the incidence of obesity and its effects when used as a preventative measure, treatment, and in the recovery process. In terms of fat and excessive weight gain, aloe can help by improving the body's metabolism, limiting the growth of fat cells, reducing the body's tendency to store fat, and improving the body's ability to create and retain muscle mass.

Through its provision of essential nutrients and amino acids, aloe vera optimizes the body's ability to process fat and protein, improving the body's synthesis of protein (building of muscle) while reducing the need for storing fat. Aloe vera also plays a role in cleansing the blood and organs of triglycerides and lipids that contribute to the storage of fat within cells and arteries. While cleansing the blood of unhealthy elements, aloe vera's effects on the cardiovascular system also help regulate blood sugar levels and minimize the risk of diabetes, a serious condition that often results from obesity.

Aloe vera is able to combat obesity by contributing essential nutrients and phytochemicals that directly impact diet, exercise, sleep, and hormone production. With an abundance of vitamins, minerals, and amino acids, aloe vera is able to provide support in the area of diet, improving the functioning of the body's systems and minimizing deficiencies that can contribute to weight gain and fatigue. The phytochemicals and enzymes that aloe contains also help regulate sleep patterns and hormone production by producing a mildly cathartic effect that can help you fall asleep and stay asleep. The elements of aloe can reduce the negative effects on weight that result from lack of sleep and erratic sleep patterns, namely the excessive production of cortisol (a weight-gain-contributing hormone) and an increased craving for carbohydrates. With the added benefits of aloe's antioxidants safeguarding the immune system from attacks that could impact health and aggravate existing conditions, aloe vera has been shown to be one of the most beneficial additions to a regimen intended to minimize obesity. Simply adding the standard recommended daily dose of 1–3 tablespoons of aloe vera to your daily diet can help to improve all of the functions involved with weight loss, management, and maintenance.

Recipes

Blueberry-Banana Breakfast Smoothie

This smoothie is a great addition to any heart-healthy diet. It's packed with antioxidants, protein, potassium, amino acids, and vitamin C to cleanse the blood, regulate blood pressure, maintain healthy blood sugar levels, and protect against illness and disease.

INGREDIENTS | SERVES 2

¼ cup aloe vera juice

¼ cup raw rolled oats

2 cups unsweetened almond milk

½ cup frozen blueberries

1 medium banana, peeled and frozen

1. Combine aloe vera and oats in a blender, and blend until oats are emulsified.

2. Add remaining ingredients and blend until all ingredients are thoroughly combined.

Almond-Blueberry Freeze

This sugar-balancing smoothie not only helps prevent diabetic conditions, but improves overall health as well.

INGREDIENTS | SERVES 2

¼ cup aloe vera juice
½ cup raw, natural unsalted almonds
1½ cups unsweetened almond milk
½ cup plain Greek yogurt
½ cup frozen blueberries

1. Combine aloe vera and almonds in a blender, and blend on high until almonds are emulsified.

2. Add remaining ingredients and blend until all ingredients are thoroughly combined.

Sweet Green Smoothie

Naturally nutrient-dense vegetables and fruit combine with antioxidant-rich green tea to help achieve and maintain optimal health at any age.

INGREDIENTS | SERVES 2

¼ cup aloe vera juice

2 cups brewed green tea, chilled

½ cup chopped spinach

½ medium pear, peeled and cored

½ medium banana, peeled and frozen

½ cup frozen blueberries

Combine all ingredients in a blender. Blend until smooth.

Pumpkin Pie Smoothie

Drinking smoothies rich in vitamin A can help improve eye health. Vitamin A is especially important to help prevent glaucoma as you age.

INGREDIENTS | SERVES 2

¼ cup aloe vera juice

½ cup pumpkin purée

½ medium sweet potato, baked and peeled

2 cups unsweetened vanilla almond milk

1 teaspoon ground cinnamon

½ teaspoon ground cloves

Combine all ingredients in a blender. Blend until smooth.

Berry-Banana Shake

The vibrant color of berries is due to the rich amounts of anthocyanins that provide powerful protection against illness and disease. With the addition of aloe and accompanying nutrient-dense foods, this smoothie takes the health benefits of berries to a whole new level, helping relieve respiratory difficulties and conditions.

INGREDIENTS | SERVES 2

¼ cup aloe vera juice

2 cups unsweetened vanilla almond milk

½ cup blackberries

½ cup raspberries

1 medium banana, peeled and frozen

Combine all ingredients in a blender. Blend until smooth.

CHAPTER 10

Inflammation

When most people hear of inflammation, they automatically think of arthritis. While arthritis is a common condition resulting from chronic inflammation, it is not the only (or even most common) condition related to inflammation. Inflammation is a natural process used by the immune system to heal the body properly, but when the normal process is disrupted, the effects are widespread throughout the body and serious health conditions can result. Luckily, aloe vera can play a major part in reducing the incidence of inflammation and its effects.

How Does Inflammation Happen?

Inflammation is not a fully understood aspect of disease, as doctors are still unsure as to the exact causes that create inflammation. Inflammation is described as an immune response that is stuck in the "on" mode. In a normal, healthy individual, inflammation is the body's response in support of the immune system; in an individual who suffers from chronic inflammation, the body's response to the trauma remains activated, causing agitation, illness, and disease.

ESSENTIAL

There are few tests for inflammation, but the medical community has identified a number of elements in the blood that are used as markers to identify people as having acute or chronic inflammation, or being predisposed to developing inflammation. With minimal tests available, most inflammation sufferers rely on self-observations and diagnoses from physicians experienced in inflammatory diseases.

When you suffer from an infection or injury, the body's response is to start the healing process as fast as possible, and support that healing process until the body returns to its normal state. At the site of an infection or injury, the body delivers pro-inflammatory agents that signal the white blood cells to begin the healing process; this part of the process, sometimes referred to as the inflammation cascade, is displayed physically with pain, redness, swelling, and heat. After the white blood cells act to clear out the infection and damaged tissues, the anti-inflammatory compounds move in to complete the healing process.

In inflammatory diseases and conditions, the activation of the pro-inflammatory compounds doesn't shut off, and the result is chronic inflammation of the area or system affected. This constant agitation leads to a domino effect of malfunctioning cells and systems throughout the body that can eventually evolve into serious inflammatory diseases that not only affect quality of life but can lead to more serious conditions.

Types of Inflammation

Inflammation can cause acute discomfort in one area or become a widespread issue plaguing one or more of the body's systems. Because it is difficult to diagnose, inflammation can progress over time and become the underlying cause of a more serious condition. With the ability to affect any tissue or cell in the body, inflammation has been identified as being the underlying cause of a number of common illnesses. While this list is short, it conveys the widespread effects that inflammation causes throughout the body, regardless of area:

- **Rheumatoid arthritis:** inflammation of the joints and tissues surrounding joints
- **Ankylosing spondylitis:** inflammation of the vertebrae, muscles, ligaments, and sacroiliac joints
- **Celiac disease:** inflammation of the small intestine
- **Crohn's disease:** inflammation of the gastrointestinal tract
- **Fibromyalgia:** inflammation of the nerves and various parts of the body
- **Graves' disease:** inflammation of the thyroid gland
- **Idiopathic pulmonary fibrosis:** inflammation of the alveoli in the lungs
- **Lupus:** inflammation of the joints, lungs, heart, kidney, and skin
- **Psoriasis:** inflammation of the skin
- **Sinusitis:** inflammation of the sinuses
- **Allergies:** inflammation of various parts of the body

With inflammation starting at a single point with just one area of the body, the spread of inflammation can result in a number of areas being plagued with the chronic condition that quickly develops into disease. Attacking the joints, nerves, muscles, ligaments, gastrointestinal tract, and bones, inflammation can impose severe limitations of the body's normal functioning and processes.

Causing stiff joints, low energy levels, inadequate digestion, skin irritations, and constant pain throughout the body, inflammation can negatively affect your overall quality of life. What's worse than suffering from mild inflammation in acute cases is the possibility of that inflammation becoming widespread. Once the inflammation of one area spreads to another, the acute evolves into chronic, and the chronic creates disease. Cancers, heart disease, and many more life-threatening conditions can arise from inflammation, and the medical treatments available rarely provide relief or reverse the condition. This is exactly why prevention may be the key to living a life without inflammation, and that is where aloe comes in.

FACT

The aloe protein, 14 kDa, was studied in depth in a recent 2010 study by Swagata Das in India; after extensive isolating and presentation of the protein to specific illnesses, the researchers concluded the aloe-specific protein to be an effective combatant against fungi and inflammation in the body. For more information, please see the information on the study in Appendix B.

Common Treatments

Inflammation can impact any part of the body and spread rapidly to other parts and systems. With inflammation being the root of these conditions and diseases, it's no wonder that billions of dollars are spent annually for treatment. Because every single person has the possibility of suffering an injury or infection at some point in her life, the possibility of developing inflammation is very real. Inflammation is a natural immune response in all humans so this worst-case scenario of suffering from an inflammation cascade that doesn't "turn off" is one that could affect any person at any time. This is exactly why the World Health Organization proposes that prevention may be the best method of treatment.

Commonly prescribed antibiotics and medications pose an equal number of risks and benefits. Nonsteroidal anti-inflammatory drugs (NSAIDs) are the widely used anti-inflammatory drug of choice. While these medications are sold over the counter, they do have long lists of possibly harmful side effects. Acetaminophen is also used in the treatment of fever and pain, but can also contribute to a host of serious issues from overuse. Prescription medications designed to block the cyclooxygenase enzyme from causing inflammation, fever, and pain may be useful and effective in the short-term, but have been linked to a higher incidence of stroke and heart disease.

ALERT

There are a growing number of physicians who are speaking out in an effort to inform consumers of the dangers of repetitive or excessive use of antibiotics. Weakening the immune system, causing adverse effects in the body and its systems, and producing an environment in which new and stronger illnesses can wreak havoc, these doctors are imploring people to use antibiotics only as a last resort.

Knowing that inflammation is part of a natural healing process, one would think the crux of the issue lies with the natural functioning of the body. Seeing the adverse effects of the commonly prescribed pharmaceutical treatments, many professionals within the health community have started questioning the treatments, suggesting the more effective way of preventing and treating this natural mishap may lie in natural methods.

Aloe vera has come into the spotlight as a treatment method for inflammation because of its natural ability to reduce inflammation while promoting the health of the body's cells and systems and improving immune system functioning (the root of inflammation). With minimal side effects, such as the laxative effect with which many aloe consumers are familiar, aloe has confirmed benefits that outweigh possible risks. With an increasing amount of research casting light on the consequences of pharmaceutical treatments, the aloe vera treatment method is growing in popularity.

How Aloe Can Help

Natural health practitioners have started implementing a more natural treatment method that focuses on targeting the root of inflammation, naturally. Having seen the negative effects of diet, inactivity, stress, sleep, and other lifestyle factors on the development and continuation of inflammation, a growing number of physicians and researchers have moved to more natural healing methods that take the entire body and it's systems into consideration.

Because of the frustration of "not knowing" the causes, effects, and effective treatment for inflammation, the medical community has joined natural practitioners, helping identify the physical conditions commonly observed in inflammation sufferers. This greater attention on the issues that may create and exacerbate inflammation, such as components of diet and lifestyle factors, has produced a vast amount of research identifying certain existing conditions that normally coincide with a diagnosis of inflammatory conditions. Luckily, this focus on the seemingly unrelated conditions associated with inflammation, coupled with a better understanding of the synergy within the body's systems, has provided possible solutions to the problem. With this turn of focus to the natural aspects of causes and effects taking place in the body suffering from inflammation, the idea that "natural conditions respond to natural treatments" is being more widely accepted for the prevention and treatment of inflammation.

FACT

In the January 2014 edition of *Carbohydrate Polymers*, Dr. Min-Cheol Kang effectively proved the aloe vera polysaccharides' (APS) free-radical-scavenging capabilities and their ability to fight off oxidative stress caused by free radicals and inflammation. For more information on the study, and how you can find out more, please see Appendix B.

When aloe was first administered for conditions of the skin and gastrointestinal system, the results were successful. Its continued use led to experimental applications of aloe in other areas of health. As time progressed and modern medicine advanced, it was determined that the naturally occurring phytochemicals in aloe provide antioxidant, antiseptic, antimicrobial, and anti-inflammatory benefits. These phytochemicals, consisting of a number of various nutrients, enzymes, and aloe-specific phytochemicals, proved to be effective in treatments then, and continue to be effective now. Providing the body with hydration, nutrition, support, and protection, aloe has shown to be beneficial in a number of areas of health, especially with inflammation. By administering aloe to an inflammation sufferer, the benefits of aloe vera's naturally occurring anti-inflammatory phytochemicals can help to correct and improve a number of systems and functions that contribute to the development and continuation of inflammation. Studies have been performed to evaluate the effectiveness of the anti-inflammatory benefits of aloe vera in every area of the body ranging from the digestive system and the skin to hemorrhoids and specific organs; the findings of these studies have shown that the use of aloe vera can contribute to the healing of inflammation and reduce the incidence of further inflammation in almost all areas of the body; for specific resources providing the studies related to aloe and its effects on inflammation, please see the appendices.

FACT

In the *International Journal of Pharmaceutics'* Issue 333 of March, 2007, a research article, "Skin permeation enhancement potential of Aloe Vera and a proposed mechanism of action based upon size exclusion and pull effect", established that aloe vera not only penetrates the skin more efficiently than similar topical applications, but also improves the ability of solutions in penetrating the skin when combined.

Amino Acids

Providing a whopping twenty of the twenty-two amino acids needed for proper system functioning of the entire body, aloe vera is able to minimize the risks and occurrence of developing inflammation. With adequate amounts of amino acids, the body's systems not only receive support, but the functions improve, immunity improves, and these two major aspects of inflammation are minimized. With arginine, isoleucine, leucine, and phenylalanine acting as powerful anti-inflammatory agents, aloe vera provides significant amounts of effective nutrients that not only minimize existing inflammation, but also act to prevent inflammation from developing. With a simple daily dose of the recommended 1–3 tablespoons of aloe vera, one can drastically improve their intake of amino acids, and experience the anti-inflammatory benefits associated with their intake and absorption.

As an added bonus, the pain that most people use over-the-counter and prescription pain medications to deal with is treated effectively and naturally by these same amino acids, sometimes proving to be more effective in pain relief than the common medications used. Supporting the immune system, these twenty amino acids not only assist by promoting proper blood flow through cardiovascular support, but also act to cleanse the blood of impurities and safeguard the body from infections caused by bacteria, viruses, fungi, and microbes, all of which would compromise the immune system and possibly lead to a chronic incidence of inflammation.

Vitamins

An astounding number of vitamins are provided from aloe vera. Vitamins A, C, E, K, and all the essential Bs work in the body to support the organs and systems, ensuring proper functioning. As you know, one vitamin deficiency can result in reduced functioning of a system, creating a domino effect in the systems that rely on the adversely affected one. Vitamins A, C, and E have been shown to contribute to the immune system's health with their antioxidant-like properties, supporting the body's immune system while maintaining proper functioning of the body's systems.

Vitamin A deficiency has been shown to be a common existing condition in inflammation sufferers; whether it be a cause or effect, addressing a vitamin A deficiency has been shown to improve the condition of inflammation, effectively reducing the inflammation and symptoms that result. Aloe vera not only provides vitamin A, but also supports the body's absorption of vitamin A by providing a number of minerals that assist in the processing and utilization of vitamins A, C, and E.

Minerals

Acting as effective multitasking support elements, minerals do double duty by supporting the body's normal functioning and also by acting as powerful electrolytes that support the health of the blood, gut, hormones, and fluid levels throughout the body. With an abundance of essential minerals like iron, magnesium, zinc, and copper that act directly on the balance of hormones, the blood's health, and the proper functioning of the cardiovascular system, it's no surprise that the minerals of aloe help relieve the condition of inflammation.

Responsible for delivering the essential nutrients to the body's organs and systems, the blood's main components, red blood cells, white blood cells, and plasma, also directly affect inflammation. The continued activation, or "calling in," of white blood cells to the site of an injury and infection is one of the precipitating factors of inflammation, which is improved when the necessary minerals help maintain proper functioning and regulation of white blood cells. The next step in the inflammatory process involves the hormones that act as pro-inflammatory agents, continuing the process and resulting in chronic inflammation. The zinc and copper that help regulate these hormones are abundant in aloe, helping improve the production and use of pro-inflammatory and anti-inflammatory hormones. Aloe vera helps minimize the improper functioning that results in the "inflammation cascade" of these hormones.

Specific Phytochemicals

Unique to aloe are a number of potent phytochemicals that work synergistically to promote health and maintain proper functioning of the body and its systems. These phytochemicals contribute to the improvement of inflammatory conditions by reducing inflammation, relieving the pain associated with inflammatory conditions, and helping regenerate tissue lost as a result of prolonged chronic inflammation.

One of these naturally occurring elements, lipase, is an enzyme that helps aloe penetrate through the skin's multiple layers when applied topically, improving the extent of the anti-inflammatory and antioxidant effects to the rest of the body and allowing those effects to reach the blood supply and, therefore all of the areas of the body that are supplied by the blood.

Helping to minimize the discomfort in all areas affected by inflammation, plant sterols such as lupeol, beta-sitosterol, and campesterol, act directly at the site of inflammation with powerful anti-inflammatory properties; these effects are not limited to the area of discomfort, though, and proceed throughout the body to seek and destroy inflammation-causing agents in the bloodstream. Reducing the pain resulting from inflamed areas of the body, aloe's salicylic acid provides an aspirin-like benefit that helps reduce pain symptoms by inhibiting the production of prostaglandin hormones that encourage inflammation and pain response in nerves. This pain-relieving aspect of aloe is accentuated by the presence of a naturally occurring enzyme, bradykinin, that helps break down powerful pain messengers that communicate between the body and the brain.

The most astounding phytochemicals provided by aloe vera in terms of inflammation prevention and treatment are the polysaccharides that actually help the tissues damaged or lost in the time of prolonged chronic inflammation regenerate and rebuild, resulting in inflammation-free areas of new cells and tissues. The generally recommended daily dosage of 1–3 tablespoons of aloe vera has shown to have beneficial effects in the reduction of inflammation, and can be improved with topical applications as well. By simply applying a generous amount of aloe vera to the inflamed areas of the body, you can reduce pain and inflammation topically, as often as necessary.

Recipes

Amazing Applesauce

This quick and easy applesauce tastes much better than the store-bought variety. The all-natural ingredients reduce inflammation in the body.

INGREDIENTS | SERVES 6

4 cups water

4 medium apples, peeled, cored, and chopped

½ cup aloe vera juice

1 teaspoon ground cinnamon

1. In a large stockpot, combine water and apples.

2. Bring to a boil over high heat. Reduce heat to low, and simmer for 30–45 minutes or until apples are fork-tender.

3. Transfer apples to a blender, and add aloe vera and cinnamon.

4. Blend on high until desired consistency is achieved.

Apple-Berry Smoothie

Satisfy your sweet tooth with this delicious anti-inflammatory drink that provides antioxidants to reduce cell damage and disease.

INGREDIENTS | SERVES 2

¼ cup aloe vera juice

2 cups unsweetened vanilla almond milk

1 medium apple, peeled, cored, and chopped

1 cup frozen strawberries

⅛ cup ground flaxseed

Combine all ingredients in a blender. Blend until smooth.

Tropical Refresher

This delightful combination of tropical tastes provides amazing health benefits to every area of the body by reducing inflammation.

INGREDIENTS | SERVES 2

¼ cup aloe vera juice

½ cup coconut oil

1½ cups water

2 cups chopped pineapple, peeled and cored

Combine all ingredients in a blender. Blend until smooth.

Simple Salsa

When a delicious food can create healthy changes in the body, it makes "eating for health" a lot easier! This splendid, slightly spicy salsa is delicious, and it also provides the entire body with vitamins, nutrients, and powerful phytochemicals!

INGREDIENTS | SERVES 10

5 small Roma tomatoes, cored and chopped

2 cloves garlic, minced

¼ cup chopped cilantro

¼ cup aloe vera juice

⅓ cup diced red onion

¼ cup diced celery

2 tablespoons lime juice

1. In a medium bowl, combine tomatoes, garlic, and cilantro, and toss to coat.

2. Add remaining ingredients and combine with a fork until all ingredients are thoroughly combined.

3. Store in the refrigerator for up to 2 days.

Roasted Turmeric Potatoes

Dense potatoes, antioxidant-rich turmeric, and healthy fats from olive oil provide blood sugar stabilization and healthy blood-fat regulation. This tasty side dish not only provides relief for those who fall victim to sugar highs and crashes, but also helps reduce chronic inflammation.

INGREDIENTS | SERVES 2

⅛ cup plus 2 tablespoons olive oil

2 large Idaho baking potatoes, peeled and cubed

1 clove garlic, minced

1 tablespoon turmeric powder

Salt and pepper, to taste

¼ cup aloe vera juice

1. Preheat oven to 400°F. Brush a large baking sheet with 2 tablespoons olive oil.

2. In a large bowl, combine potatoes, remaining olive oil, garlic, and turmeric. Pour potatoes onto baking sheet and spread out evenly.

3. Bake for 20 minutes, or until fork-tender. Toss to turn and continue baking for 15 minutes, or until all potatoes are lightly browned.

4. Remove from oven and sprinkle with salt and pepper. Cool for 5 minutes before tossing with aloe vera to coat.

CHAPTER 11

Brain Health

The brain is the most complex organ of the entire body, responsible for the messages, actions, and functioning of every system of the body. Supported by the nutrients that affect the systems and the components that act to directly service those systems, the brain is the main control system from which every part of the body receives direction. From actions and reactions to thought and creativity, the brain is the powerhouse of the body from which all orders are given. With all the power it holds, the brain's malfunctioning can pose major problems for the mental and physical processes we hold as normal "day-to-day" functions. With the current knowledge about the needs and responsibilities of the brain, we can take necessary steps to improve and maintain brain health and proper brain functioning.

Aloe vera is one of the additions to everyday life that can provide major benefits in the maintenance of brain health, reversing damage and making improvements for years to come.

An Introduction to Your Brain

By far, the brain is the most complex and powerful organ in the body. This three-pound organ is divided into two hemispheres, three main functioning areas, three lobes, and a number of supporting structures that act as communication delivery systems from the brain to the body (and vice versa). With a simple breakdown of the aspects of the brain and a brief overview of each component's function, you can better understand how synergistically this organ functions, and the importance of maintaining proper health of the body's supporting systems to ensure proper functioning of the brain as a whole. With millions of reactions taking place in the brain every second, it's easy to understand how a minor malfunction can cause major complications. Not like a cascade or domino effect as seen in other aspects of the body's health, a problem in the brain leads to a direct issue of corresponding parts of the body with either a deterioration of activity and communication or complete inactivity.

Able to manage, control, and coordinate an astounding number of actions, reactions, functions, processes, and system synergy, the brain is made up of interactive parts, supporting subsections, and essential elements that combine to make breathing, respiration, digestion, movement, thought, and emotions possible. With just one area adversely affected, the remaining areas falter, leading to disruptions in thought, memory, behavior, speech, learning, etc. By being informed about the parts of the brain, and how each of those parts contributes to our everyday functioning, you can better understand the importance of brain health and how to better support those areas to safeguard and optimize your own brain's functioning.

Two Hemispheres

The brain is divided into two hemispheres, left and right. With every structural component, there is a left and a right, mirroring one another and supporting the functioning of different aspects of the body. A surprising fact is that as the messages from the brain to the body (and vice versa) communicate, their messages crisscross. In other words, the left brain and right body communicate while the right brain and left body communicate; this is displayed in a stroke sufferer who has had a stroke on the left side of the brain and is unable to control the right side of the body, and vice versa. These two hemispheres are further separated into three areas.

Each of the three areas of the brain is located at different geological points of the brain and controls different aspects of normal functions, and communicates with different systems. These three areas are the hindbrain, midbrain, and forebrain, and are responsible for the body's healthy functioning in different ways:

- The **hindbrain** is located in the back of the brain, and includes the upper spinal cord, brain stem, and cerebellum. The hindbrain is responsible for body functions like heart rate, respiratory functioning, and digestion, the innate functions of the body that do not require conscious control.
- Set at the uppermost portion of the brainstem, the **midbrain** controls reflex actions and is involved in voluntary movements such as eye movements.
- The **forebrain** is the largest and most developed portion of the brain, consisting of the cerebrum, thalamus, and hypothalamus. Also referred to as the "inner brain," the forebrain processes and utilizes information, communicating the information to the rest of the brain and the body. The cerebral cortex is the part of the brain responsible for thought, behavior, and action. It is the cerebral cortex that is further broken down into four different sections, called lobes.

Four Lobes

The four lobes of the cerebral cortex each control different functions throughout the body. Processing information about sights and smells, information and education, visual recognition, memory formation, etc., these lobes are the mini control centers of the brain that are responsible for different aspects of one's self. Impacting one of these lobes can completely alter an individual's personality, memory, ability to speak, thought processing, and ability to control physical functions. With such important roles, these four lobes are discussed at length when the brain and its functions are presented:

- **Frontal lobe:** responsible for planning, imagination, reasoning, speech, emotions, and problem solving, the frontal lobe is essential for the formation of great ideas and heated debates.
- **Parietal lobe:** set behind the frontal lobe, this lobe is responsible for recognition, movement, orientation, and processing information of the senses. The taste, textures, and smells of an amazing meal are all developed here, as well as the physical control that allows you to cut and move food to your mouth using intricate movements with your knife, fork, or spoon.
- **Occipital lobe:** set behind the eyes, the occipital lobe is responsible for processing visual information. The beauty of fall leaves, a sunset, and rainbows are all captured and related by this lobe.
- **Temporal lobe:** this lobe is responsible for perception, emotion, recognition, auditory information processing, memory, and speech. The song that you heard when you were eighteen that made you cry is stored as a memory here.

Supporting Components

With all the activity in the brain dictating and supporting every aspect of life, the components that support the brain's functioning play crucial roles. The cells, neurons, and synapses that make up the actual matter of the brain also serve as communication pathways between different cells of the brain's structures and between the brain and the body's systems. With a malfunction of just one area of these supporting structures, the entire body is affected.

- **Neurons:** these mini powerhouses create messages that are carried via neurotransmitters at speeds of 400 miles per hour to and from other neurons, "speaking" to the brain and body about movement, thoughts, feelings, and memories. Within and just outside the neuron are specialized structures that not only serve a purpose for the neuron, but also support the communication between the neurons and the brain-body connection.

- **Cell body:** containing the nucleus, the cell body manufactures energy molecules to support the functioning of the neuron.
- **Dendrites:** extending like branches from the cell body, the dendrites are responsible for bringing messages to the cell.
- **Axons:** reaching out from the cell body much like the dendrites, axons are responsible for the process of carrying messages away from the cell body. The axons trigger the release of neurotransmitters into the synapses, carrying messages to the receptors located within the corresponding cells, organs, and systems.
- **Sheath:** not just a protective layer for the neuron, the myelin sheath serves to encourage speed of message sending and receiving. Promoting the health of the neuron's myelin sheath ensures that the optimal speed, estimated to be about 400 miles per hour, is possible.

With the functions of each of these elements being thoroughly dependent on one another, it's easy to see how simple malfunctions or deteriorations in the health of just one element can create disastrous effects in the functioning of the entire body. Maintaining the health of these supporting structures of the brain is crucial in maintaining brain health and the health of the body with which it communicates. Studies have shown that these components of the brain thrive with adequate supplies of oxygen, macronutrients, micronutrients, and a steady amount of glucose.

With aloe's ability to help support and regulate blood sugar levels, supply a number of vitamins and minerals that are needed for proper functioning and processing within cells, and improve the body's processing of the oxygen supply to the brain, it's easy to see that regular consumption of aloe can help maintain the health of the very components that directly affect the health of the brain.

Dysfunctions of the Brain

The National Institute of Neurological Disorders and Stroke conduct and support hundreds of studies on the brain and its functioning every year. Since the 1990s the amount of information about the brain, its systems, and its functions has become clearer due to countless researchers and studies throughout the world. Many of these studies have focused on the functioning of the normal brain, giving us insight into the processes, needs, and symbiotic relations on which the brain depends in order to function at its best. Conversely, many of these studies have been on brains suffering from degeneration, trauma, or disease, resulting in malfunctioning in the brain's processes. These malfunctions have been organized into categories that classify dysfunctions by their cause, area affected, or symptoms that are produced as a result of the dysfunction:

- **Neurogenetic:** faulty genes are responsible for the development of neurological disorders such as Huntington's disease and muscular dystrophy.
- **Developmental:** in the process of development, dysfunctions can occur within any area of the brain and spinal cord leading to conditions such as spinal bifida.
- **Degenerative:** as one ages, a deterioration of the brain and its components leads to the damage or death of essential nerve cells, resulting in degenerative disorders such as Parkinson's and Alzheimer's disease.
- **Metabolic:** as a result of improper metabolic functioning, the brain functioning is affected and results in conditions such as Gaucher's disease.
- **Cerebrovascular:** diseases that affect the blood vessels supplying the brain with necessary oxygen and blood create complications in the brain's functioning and result in conditions such as strokes and vascular dementia.
- **Trauma:** an injury to the brain or spinal cord can seriously impact the brain's functioning and the nerves that assist in the communication between the brain and body. Paralysis is just one example of how damage to the brain or spinal cord can lead to complete "disconnection" between the brain and body.
- **Convulsive:** epilepsy and epileptic experiences result in seizures, the physical manifestation of brain and body malfunctioning.
- **Infectious:** bacteria, viruses, and inflammation can severely impact the health of the brain and spinal cord, resulting in infections and serious damage to the cells and areas of the nervous system. AIDS, dementia, meningitis, and encephalitis are just a few conditions that result from infection and inflammation within the nervous system.
- **Cancerous:** the development of abnormal cells within the brain can inhibit overall brain functioning or remain specific to one area of the

brain. As a result of this cancerous growth, tumors and disease can ravage the brain's cells and result in dysfunction or death.

Maintaining Brain Health

Modern technology has enabled researchers to learn more about the brain in the past two decades than in any century prior. With imagery and observations, the medical community has been able to better understand the areas of the brain, their functions and dysfunctions, their needs, and the consequences of improper care. In order to maintain brain health, numerous lifestyle choices and activities come into play to work synergistically in directly improving the health of the brain while also improving the health of the systems that support it. Through diet, mental activity, physical activity, and lifestyle choices that can minimize stress, illness, and exposure to harmful elements, the brain can not only function properly, it can thrive!

Diet

With so many areas and processes of the brain requiring a number of essential nutrients in order to function properly, it is imperative to maintain a healthy diet that supplies these essentials in adequate amounts. Requiring amino acids, glucose, vitamins, minerals, and antioxidants from the food consumed, every component and function of the brain relies on nutrition delivered through diet. With nutritional deficiencies directly impacting brain health and the functioning of every system of the body, a focus on healthy nutrition not only improves and maintains the health of the brain, but the entire body as a whole.

Physical Activity

"A body in motion stays in motion" doesn't just refer to the muscles and joints. By regularly engaging in physical activity, the brain-body connection remains engaged. Through continued use, the cells and systems that work synergistically to produce movement and communicate back and forth stimulate the brain's cells to fire, and the more those stimuli are presented, the better the brain remains capable of reacting and responding. With physical activity, the brain releases endorphins that create feelings of excitement and improve overall mood; these feelings lead to a greater desire to foster health, improving the chances of engaging in physical activity and perpetuating a cycle of continued healthy habits that all contribute to the health of the brain and the body.

Lifestyle Choices

Whether the cause is stress or exposure to harmful environmental elements, the brain suffers from certain lifestyle choices. Exposure to adverse elements such as aluminum and mercury (just to name a couple of the countless harmful elements) can have a serious impact on the brain's components and its processes, inhibiting the natural processes that take place in the brain and body. With an increasing amount of information on the impact of stress on the brain, it is now widely accepted that trauma and situations that create stress can not only affect mood, but have the capability of causing physical damage to the structural components of the brain. With possible results such as a reduction in the production of hormones, compromised processes that are involved in communication, and the development of serious illnesses and diseases, the lifestyle factors that expose the brain and body to harmful elements (both physical and psychological) should be eliminated in order to maintain the health of the brain.

How Aloe Can Help

For thousands of years, aloe has been used to treat ailments, but not until recently was there information available about how aloe can help improve the functioning and maintain the health of the brain. With countless studies and research, aloe has been shown to make remarkable improvements throughout the body and, especially, the brain. Through its provision of the necessary nutrients required by the brain, aloe is able to support the different parts of the brain, its processes, and its communication to every cell and system of the body. With specific phytochemicals that help fight disease, prevent inflammation, and cleanse the blood, aloe not only supports the brain's health, but also protects it and the systems on which it relies.

Glucose

Depending on a steady amount of readily supplied glucose, the brain's highly metabolic functions and processes rely on the body's ability to produce and regulate the amount of glucose in the blood. Providing the cells with the fuel needed to produce energy, glucose directly affects the functions of the brain's cells; with proper cell functioning, the brain is able to produce the millions of reactions that occur every second, making physical movements, thoughts, and emotions possible. With insufficient glucose available, or hypoglycemia, the brain suffers on a cellular level, resulting in lack of concentration, reduced reaction time, and fatigue.

Aloe helps in the processing and regulation of glucose not only through its ability to stabilize blood sugars, but also by providing the numerous nutrients needed to metabolize glucose and make it available to the cells for use. With B vitamins, amino acids, and all minerals required for the processing of glucose, aloe directly promotes the healthy functioning of the brain's cells and supports the processes with which they're involved.

Amino Acids

These acids that are involved in every reaction in the body are needed most in the brain. In order to create and support the neurotransmitters that are responsible for carrying the millions of messages to and from the brain's cells, the brain needs ample amounts of amino acids.

Providing twenty of the twenty-two amino acids, aloe is able to ensure the brain has the necessary amount of aminos to produce new neurotransmitters and maintain the health of the existing ones. Further supporting the use of amino acids in the production of neurotransmitters, aloe's healthy supplies of zinc work to ensure the processing of the amino acids works correctly and promotes the functioning of the newly synthesized neurotransmitters that result from the process.

Vitamins

Aloe provides the body with all the essential B vitamins, which help the brain in its production of the myelin sheath that surrounds neurons. With this protective coating helping to ensure the quick occurrence of chemical reactions and fast delivery of electrical impulses, the brain and the body rely heavily on the quality of this essential coating. Aloe vera's unique provision of these vitamins (it is the only plant that contains B_{12}) helps ensure the quality of the myelin sheath's production and development.

Another essential B vitamin provided by aloe is thiamin, which is used by the brain to maintain the membranes of brain cells and improve the conductivity of nerves. An added benefit of aloe's rich vitamin B provisions is the regulation of a byproduct of amino acid metabolism called homocysteine; by providing B_6, B_{12}, and folate required for the regulation of homocysteine levels, aloe helps prevent brain degeneration that leads to disorders like cognitive dysfunction and Alzheimer's that are caused by excessive levels of homocysteine.

In addition to the B vitamins, the brain needs ample amounts of vitamin C in order to create the norepinephrine that acts as a neurotransmitter. Not only is this vitamin supplied by aloe, but the many minerals that are also found in aloe help increase the body's absorption of vitamin C, making it more readily available for use by the brain.

Minerals

Minerals are used by the brain, not only to support the production and development of its components, but also as supportive nutrients that help in maintenance. Promoting the proper functioning of the brain's cells and the neurotransmitters that communicate the messages between them, minerals are essential in maintaining the health of the brain's inner components and the physical and psychological processes those components affect.

Calcium promotes the production of neurotransmitters and supports the system by which they are released from the neuron. Aloe's provision of this mineral helps maintain proper communication between the brain and the body.

Iron supports the production of the essential myelin sheath that improves the delivery of messages between neurons and cells; by providing iron, aloe not only maintains the proper functioning of this process, but also improves the health of the blood, helping the cardiovascular system's efficient delivery of blood, oxygen, and nutrients to the brain.

Zinc is another necessary brain-health nutrient provided by aloe that helps the cellular processes related to attention, learning, and memory, reducing the incidence of degenerative disorders. Playing a crucial role in the enzymatic reactions that make muscle control (both voluntary and involuntary) possible, magnesium is just one more mineral provided by aloe that helps improve the brain's processes and maintain overall health and quality of life.

Phytochemicals

In addition to providing the nutrients that are needed for all processes related to the brain, aloe contains a number of powerful phytochemicals that improve the brain's functioning and safeguard its health. The antioxidants provided by aloe help fight cellular malformations that lead to cancer growth and impede the functioning of the inner workings of the brain. With antibacterial, antiviral, and antimicrobial properties, aloe vera also acts to reduce the risk of infection within the brain by cleansing the blood (the delivery system that supplies the brain) and the cells of the brain and body of infectious germs, bacteria, and viruses.

One of aloe's most helpful benefits for maintaining brain health comes from its naturally occurring polysaccharides. Polysaccharides help regenerate cells and tissue that have experienced damage from inflammation and support the health of existing cells and tissues responsible for every thought, action, and process that is controlled by the brain.

Recipes

Coconut Oil Coffee

This popular combination of medium-chain fatty-acid-containing coconut oil and caffeinated coffee is not only stimulating, but beneficial to the brain and body too.

INGREDIENTS | SERVES 2

12 ounces hot brewed caffeinated coffee

½ cup aloe vera juice

2 tablespoons pure coconut oil

1. Combine coffee, aloe vera, and coconut oil in a blender with the opening adjusted to allow heat to be released.

2. Blend on high until coffee is frothy and turns a light brown.

3. Pour and enjoy!

Dark Cherry Dream

This cleansing, craving-curbing smoothie packs a punch with
vitamins and minerals that improve brain functioning.

INGREDIENTS | SERVES 2

¼ cup aloe vera juice

2 cups unsweetened vanilla almond milk

½ cup pitted cherries

½ cup pitted dates

½ medium banana, peeled and frozen

½ teaspoon ground cinnamon

Combine all ingredients in a blender. Blend until smooth.

Great Guacamole

With powerful antioxidants that help protect against illness, disease, and cancerous changes within the entire body's cells, this delicious dip is a brain- and body-protecting snack that can be enjoyed anytime.

INGREDIENTS | SERVES 2

¼ cup aloe vera juice

2 medium Hass avocados, peeled and pitted

1 tablespoon lime juice

½ cup diced red onion

¼ cup diced celery

½ cup diced tomato

2 tablespoons lime juice

1. Combine aloe vera and avocados in a medium bowl and mash until combined but still chunky.

2. Add remaining ingredients and toss together with a fork until ingredients are thoroughly combined.

3. Store in the refrigerator for up to 2 days. Cover with plastic wrap that touches the entire surface of the guacamole to prevent oxidizing.

Banana-Nut Smoothie

This combination of delicious ingredients provides essential vitamins, minerals, and amino acids while boosting brain health with the provision of omegas and antioxidants.

INGREDIENTS | SERVES 2

¼ cup aloe vera juice
½ cup chopped walnuts
2 cups unsweetened vanilla almond milk
1 medium banana, peeled and frozen
½ teaspoon ground cloves
½ teaspoon ground cinnamon

1. Combine aloe vera and walnuts in a blender, and blend on high until walnuts are emulsified.

2. Add remaining ingredients, and blend until all ingredients are thoroughly combined.

Spicy Coffee Smoothie

Caffeine improves cognitive functioning, focus, and attention, and naturally occurring phytochemicals provide protection against illness in this spicy wake-up smoothie.

INGREDIENTS | SERVES 2

¼ cup aloe vera juice

1 cup unsweetened vanilla almond milk

1½ cups brewed caffeinated coffee, chilled

⅛ teaspoon ground cayenne pepper

1 teaspoon organic maple syrup

Combine all ingredients in a blender. Blend until smooth.

CHAPTER 12

Aloe Vera Benefits for Children

From the time that conception occurs, every element within a child's environment plays a role in development. It is now known that particular nutrients play a major role in the development of a child's body, brain, and even personality, and those nutrients can either help or hinder proper growth. Surprisingly, the addition of aloe vera can not only help the body's processing and utilization of the essential nutrients needed for health, but can also help promote optimal functioning of all the body's processes and safeguard the child's health as well!

From Conception to Birth

Even before conception, the biological factors that play major roles in the proper development of an embryo, and then the fetus, make huge differences in the outcome of the physical, psychological, and emotional growth of a child. Before birth, the adequate nutrients required for the production of cells, nerves, and glands must be present in order to ensure proper development and system functioning. With adequate supplies of macronutrients and micronutrients in utero, the health of a child can be optimized not only before birth, but also throughout every year of development after birth.

With aloe vera having the ability to optimize the absorption of nutrients, and further improve the functioning of the body's systems in order to promote better use of those nutrients, it's no surprise that aloe is being studied and researched to determine the safety and efficiency of adding aloe vera to a prenatal routine. As with all new implementations that occur during pregnancy, one should always consult their physician before adding aloe vera to your daily routine.

ALERT

Chickenpox is a virus that is reported throughout the world, and is most commonly seen among children ages five through ten. While the virus runs its course and resolves itself naturally, the topical use of aloe vera on the skin can help to alleviate pain and minimize inflammation associated with the skin irritation caused by the virus.

Vitamins

The vitamins required by a growing fetus are exhaustive. From A through E, every single one of the vitamins is needed in order to ensure a fetus's proper development. With a deficiency in just one vitamin, the results can be catastrophic. Spina bifida is just one physical malformation that can result from inadequate intake and utilization of B vitamins; improper growth and enclosure of the spine results in physical deformation that can plague a baby with pain and suffering for life. Ensuring a baby receives each essential vitamin through the expectant mom's diet and supplementation, a baby can thrive throughout pregnancy and well into life.

B Vitamins

B vitamins play major roles in the development of the brain's cells, nerves, and connections, while also maintaining the health of the growing spine. The blood, bones, brain, and even the body's proper system functioning all begin with B vitamins in utero. Responsible for the development of eyesight, hormone production, and the future development of teeth, all the B vitamins are needed in ample supplies throughout pregnancy.

Vitamins A, C, and E

With vitamins A, C, and E playing synergistic roles that help one another in fostering a baby's sound development, the bones, nerves, and blood all benefit from the adequate intake of these essential vitamins. Further improving the health of a child throughout pregnancy and beyond, these vitamins also improve the development of a strong immune system, while protecting the unborn baby from illnesses and diseases that can hinder proper growth and development in utero.

ALERT

The World Health Organization estimates that approximately 250 million preschool aged children are vitamin A deficient. Without proper nutrition, this deficiency can lead to disastrous consequences; every year, 250,000–500,000 children lose their sight as a result of vitamin A deficiency.

Minerals

The minerals needed throughout pregnancy not only ensure that the mom's body remains healthy and able to carry and deliver a healthy baby, but also provide the support needed for the development of the baby. From conception through birth, ample supplies of minerals are needed in order to ensure that the fetus is able to process nutrients and develop properly.

Calcium

While most people associate calcium with building and maintaining strong bones, this mineral actually assists in far more than just bone development in utero. Responsible for the growth and formation of the skeletal system and teeth, an adequate supply of calcium is also needed for the development of nerves and the support of their functioning, as well as the health of the blood. Without essential calcium supplies, the placenta is unable to provide the growing fetus with the nutrients needed for growth, and can even lead to the development of blood clots.

Iron

A baby's development of hemoglobin begins in utero, and iron plays a major role in that development. Not only ensuring that the blood has all necessary components, iron supplies reduce the chances of anemia and can minimize the risk of low birth weight and premature delivery.

Zinc

A major brain requirement, zinc is responsible for promoting the growth and development of the brain and each of its components. Ensuring the proper communication between each element of the brain, zinc helps promote the proper development and functioning of nerves, cells, and pathways responsible for motor control, speech development, and cognition. Also required for the production and processing of insulin and essential enzymatic activities, zinc is an essential mineral that is required throughout every step of development.

ALERT

Protein is a valuable nutrient needed by all children, helping to promote the proper growth and development of everything from the brain to the body's systems. Children between the ages of one and eight require an average of 13–19 grams of protein daily, while children and adolescents between the ages of nine and eighteen require between 34–52 grams per day.

How Aloe Can Help

Throughout pregnancy, the needs and requirements of an expectant mother and her fetus ebb and flow. With adequate supplies of each vitamin and mineral being provided through diet and supplementation, mom and baby can grow as intended without issue. Aloe can not only help the intake of the essential vitamins and minerals needed for pregnancy with its own supplies of each necessary nutrient, but can also help by promoting the proper system development and functioning that delivers and utilizes those nutrients, all while increasing the availability of the nutrients consumed. Aloe's unique phytochemicals enable the mom-to-be and baby to benefit from increased absorption of vitamins and minerals, making both less likely to experience deficiencies throughout pregnancy and after birth. As an added benefit for the pregnancy experience, the use of aloe has not only been shown to reduce the incidence of nausea, but can also help maintain proper electrolyte balance within both mom and baby, reducing risks associated with dehydration that can result from morning sickness.

Illness and Disease Prevention

Children are exposed to a number of microbes, bacteria, and viruses that can result in illnesses and disease. With immune systems that are less developed and efficient than adults, children are more likely to succumb to illness through exposure to people, places, and things that would rarely affect well-developed immune systems. Further complicating the immunity issue, children are often exposed to one another in enclosed areas like classrooms while engaged in play; germs in the air and on surfaces are quickly shared among the children, and can be transmitted throughout a group even when no symptoms are displayed. In order to combat the contraction of illness, a focus on immunity is a must for any child, birth through adolescence.

Immunity

Vitamin C has long been known as a strong immunity-boosting prevention and cure against illness. Because this powerful vitamin plays a major role in building the body's defenses, it is by far one of the most important nutrients available to improve the body's immune system. The full spectrum of vitamins and minerals, as well as ample supplies of proteins, carbohydrates, and fats, are necessary to support the body's proper functioning, and when a deficiency occurs that results in an imbalance or impaired system functioning, the body's defenses can also be impaired. With diet and supplementation ensuring the body has what it needs to function properly, the immune system can not only work as intended, but also utilize specialized nutrients that act as powerful protectants to improve the body's defenses even further.

FACT

Children need vitamin C for proper growth and development, but also for the maintenance of a healthy immune system capable of fending off illness and disease. The daily recommendation of vitamin C for children is between 15–25 mg for children ages one to eight, and 45–75 mg for children and adolescents nine through eighteen years of age.

With aloe vera's unique combination of specialized phytochemicals, the support it is able to provide to the immune system moves far beyond the functioning experienced with simple dietary recommendations. Powerful antioxidants not only help prevent against infection, but also assist the body in maintaining clean and healthy blood and prevent against dangerous unhealthy changes on the cellular level. Reserving the body's ability to focus on the everyday needs of the body and its systems, aloe vera acts to prevent illness while promoting health.

Bacterial Infections

Exposure to bacteria is an everyday occurrence. In a child's daily life, this normal exposure can wreak havoc on an already overwhelmed immune system. With an immature immune system that is focused on ridding the body of microbes that are inhaled and absorbed throughout the average day, children are extremely susceptible to developing a bacterial infection. Whether the infection takes hold of the skin, airways, or blood, bacterial infections can quickly develop into colds, festering wounds, or serious illnesses. While proper hygiene and frequently washing hands throughout the day can minimize the risk of bacterial infections, aloe can help reduce the risk even further.

With powerful phytochemicals that act as antibacterial agents, aloe is able to purge the blood of bacteria and reduce the risk of exposure to the bacteria throughout the body. By helping fend off the infection caused by bacterial exposure both internally and externally, aloe vera has shown to be effective in ridding the skin, blood, and even respiratory system of harmful bacteria that can otherwise develop into serious illnesses. Supported by the antioxidants of the vitamins A, C, and E that are provided by aloe, this simple addition to the immunity-boosting regimen can effectively safeguard the health of the body's cells and systems while preventing the spread of infection.

Viral Infections

Flus and viruses can be harmful and debilitating in adults, but in children, viruses can be downright deadly. Since there are few medicinal treatments available that can combat viruses, viral infections are best treated with prevention. Healthy immunity is absolutely necessary in minimizing the risk of contracting a virus, and a healthy immunity can reduce the severity and duration of a viral infection as well. With a diet consisting of healthy fruit and vegetables that are rich in essential immunity-boosting nutrients, an immune system can function as intended and help protect against viruses and their infections. The vitamins A, C, and E, as well as the minerals iron and zinc, can help protect against viruses by supporting the immune system and by ensuring that the essential nutrients needed for protection are available. The absorption of these essential viral-fighting vitamins and minerals is improved by the use of aloe vera.

Aloe vera is able to further support the immunity against viruses by providing antiviral agents that bind with viral infections in the body. Whether the infection is on the skin or attempting to take hold internally, aloe vera's antiviral phytochemicals not only help remove the infectious virus, but also help improve the body's defenses. Topically and internally, aloe's antiviral agents can help prevent a virus from taking hold, while aloe's provisions of immunity-boosting nutrients further support the immune system and promote its functioning. This one-two punch of prevention and protection helps reduce the risk of viral infections that can take hold in any organ, tissue, or system, helping to protect a child from contracting a virus, and minimizing the severity of a virus that may have already been introduced. The recommendation for children's consumption of aloe vera varies, but is generally considered safe in the amount of ½–1 tablespoon daily; this amount can be gradually increased as the child progresses through adolescence. The child's daily dose of aloe vera can provide immunity-boosting preventative nutrients and phytochemicals that can assist the body in fighting off viruses, and this dose can be doubled while a child is suffering from a virus and its symptoms. The daily dose consumed by teens on a regular basis can also be doubled during periods of sickness, returning to the original daily dose after the illness has subsided.

Serious Disease

Children are not immune from the serious diseases that plague adults. With inadequate immune system functioning, the body's cells can change from healthy to diseased. Optimizing the immune system and protecting the body against these dangerous changes is crucial in safeguarding a child's health and development. With the antibacterial and antiviral agents that act to protect against infection and provide support for the immune system, aloe vera not only provides support for the very systems that safeguard health, but can also reduce the risk of changes at the cellular level. Powerful antioxidants that protect against infection can also help maintain cell health and reduce the incidence of cellular changes that set off disease and illness. With ample supplies of the vitamins and minerals needed to provide this support, aloe vera also provides the antioxidants thought to improve cell health and system functioning, helping to prevent serious illness and disease.

Proper Growth and Development

Children require proper nutrition to ensure the proper growth and development of everything from the brain and bones to digestive system and hormone production. Because the body consists of synergistic systems that depend on one another for support, a deficiency in even one nutrient can result in a domino effect that resounds in multiple areas of development.

The most common deficiencies seen in children are those relating to vitamin D, B vitamins, and iron, but the symptoms that result from nutrient deficiencies are alarmingly similar to the common ailments reported by children and their parents. ADHD, slow speech development, chronic fatigue, impaired cognitive development, frequent illnesses, etc., can all be traced back to severe deficiencies of vitamins and nutrients.

Aloe vera is able to help ensure the proper growth and development of a child in a number of ways. With bountiful provisions of essential nutrients and the added benefit of improved absorption of nutrients, aloe vera is also able to help by ensuring the body's systems are functioning properly and remain free of problematic health issues that can result in developmental disasters.

Hormones and Growth

The pituitary gland is responsible for hormone production and secretion throughout the body. A dysfunction of this hormone can lead to slow metabolism, impaired growth, insulin-related issues, and delayed puberty. Not surprisingly, the nutritional needs for the proper functioning of the pituitary gland are often neglected in today's standard American diet. Vitamin E, and the minerals manganese and magnesium, help support the proper functioning of the pituitary gland and the production of the hormones necessary for proper growth; these nutrients are commonly found in leafy greens and whole fruit and vegetables, and can be consumed in adequate amounts simply through a balanced diet. Aloe vera not only ensures that these much-needed nutrients are available, but it further supports the production and dispersion of those hormones by improving the cardiovascular system and nerve communication that relays the signals between the pituitary gland and the body. Through the improved functioning of the neurons that results from the phytochemicals contained in aloe vera, the brain and all of the body's systems are able to communicate more efficiently; this results in improved hormone production and regulation, cognitive functioning, and mental clarity.

Cognitive Development

With a number of factors that combine to provide children with all things related to thought, emotion, and mood, the brain is one area of health that should take precedence for growth and development. The brain acts as a control center that can direct a child's development not only physically, but psychologically and emotionally as well. With aloe vera's provisions of B vitamins, and the additional amino acids and nutrients that improve B-vitamin absorption, a number of brain activities improve, including the regulation and improvement of emotions and mood.

Mood and Depression

While there are a number of opinions that suggest that pharmaceutical treatments can help improve bouts of depression, anxiety, attention disorders, and so on, it can help to understand that ample supplies of the nutrients that support brain health can optimize the functioning of the processes controlled by the brain and conversely, deficiencies of those essential nutrients can result in malfunctioning. One of the main groups of nutrients that have been associated with happiness and depression are those of the B variety. Because the B vitamins play major roles in the development of "feel good" hormones like serotonin and dopamine, and also contribute to the proper development and functioning of the nerve cells in the brain, the amount of B vitamins consumed in the diet can impact the stability of mood and help alleviate bouts of depression.

Aloe vera provides B vitamins and essential nutrients that combine to support brain health, nervous system functioning, and communication within the brain and between the brain and body. Aloe vera has been shown to improve depression, reduce anxiety, improve cognitive functioning, and minimize stress among children. The essential nutrients that are provided by aloe vera also help improve cardiovascular health and blood quality, which can contribute to healthier system functioning and minimize the risk of elevated blood pressure, often associated with elevated anxiety levels, disruptions in thought processes, and higher incidences of stress. The recommended daily dose of ½–1 tablespoon of aloe vera can provide a child with benefits relating to mood and emotional well-being. Teens are able to consume a gradually increased daily dose between 1–2 tablespoons of aloe vera for improved mood benefits.

Skeletal and Muscle Development

The crucial stores and supplies of essential nutrients are imperative for the proper growth of the skeleton and muscular systems of every growing child. Minerals like calcium, iron, magnesium, manganese, and many more are utilized by the body to provide the framework and support in the development of bones and tissues, while numerous vitamins and essential nutrients further promote the proper functioning of this developmental process. The muscular system also depends on the dietary intake of vitamins, minerals, and macronutrients in order to develop properly, helping to form and maintain the muscle mass that provides the support for the skeletal system. These two systems work together to provide the support a growing body needs in order to sit, stand, move, and play. With deficiencies of crucial nutrients, though, these two systems suffer and wreak havoc on the body and life of a developing child; in times of need, the stores of calcium get depleted from bones and the body can turn to existing muscle mass when in need of protein and amino acids. Helping to improve the body's ability to absorb and maintain proper stores of essential bone- and muscle-building nutrients, a healthy diet rich in whole foods that provide essential micronutrients and macronutrients needed for bone and muscle health can be made more efficient through the simple addition of aloe. The recommended daily dose of ½–1 tablespoon of aloe vera can provide a child with nutritive benefits, optimizing growth and development, and teens are able to consume a gradually increased daily dose between 1–2 tablespoons of aloe vera.

Nutrition

Without a doubt, nutrition plays a major role in the overall functioning of the body. Without adequate supplies of the body's required nutrients, deficiencies and dysfunctions result. For children, the effects are far more serious because the deficiencies and upsets in the diet not only cause problems in childhood, but can spell disaster for a lifetime as well. In order to maintain optimal health, a focus on nutrition surpasses the body's basic needs and can help prevent a number of dangerous health issues that can adversely affect the life of a developing child.

Many children who regularly consume the standard American diet (accurately referred to by its acronym, SAD) filled with sodium, sugar, and refined carbohydrates battle with common illnesses and disease that impair their body's systems and limit their abilities throughout life. From obesity and diabetes to respiratory complications and allergies, the results of malnutrition can create complications that affect quality of life.

Obesity

One out of every three children under the age of eighteen is now considered overweight or obese. With these staggering statistics, pediatricians are turning their focus from recommendations that primarily encouraged more exercise to an emphasis on better nutrition. Without proper nutrition, a child lacks the energy and physical ability to engage in exercise, creating barriers that lead to a cycle of less physical activity and more profound effects of malnutrition that further compound weight-related issues. With the positive results of a nutritious diet having shown to improve every area of physical and mental health, the focus on nutrition in children is one that is well supported.

With a daily diet that includes whole foods, the body is able to function properly and better regulate every physical and mental function, minimizing the risks associated with malnutrition. Not surprisingly, aloe vera's components have been shown to further support a nutritious diet, improve energy levels, and assist in each of the body's systems that are involved in maintaining proper health and optimal functioning.

Diabetes

Type 1 and type 2 diabetes are insulin-related diseases that can lead to serious complications and limitations in the life of a child. Whether the disease is genetic (type 1) or developed (type 2), a nutritious diet that focuses on improving the body's ability to regulate insulin and maintain blood health is crucial. Once referred to as adult-onset diabetes, type 2 diabetes is now being diagnosed in children at younger ages every year. For example, there were no children diagnosed with this disease in 1980, and an estimated 60,000 diagnosed in 2012. With this growing problem, the focus on prevention and treatment of type 2 diabetes is now being addressed by pediatricians and placing a growing responsibility on parents. Processed foods packed with excessive sugars are being provided to today's children for every meal and snack, and the result can be catastrophic in the fragile, developing system of a child. A combination of sound nutrition, regular exercise, and aloe vera can help avoid the onset of diabetes and minimize the complications that arise as a result. While a physician should be consulted before the implementation of a new natural or medicinal addition to a diabetic lifestyle, the general recommendation for aloe vera consumption would be ½–1 tablespoon daily for children, gradually increasing to a daily dose of 1–2 tablespoons of aloe vera for teens.

By helping the body to process foods, maintain clean blood, and regulate the amount of glucose in the bloodstream, aloe vera is able to assist the body's every process related to digestion, nutrient processing, and blood sugar regulation. These benefits directly improve the health and well-being of a child, improving the precise processes that are related to diabetes. With added benefits that improve immunity, optimize system functioning, and improve the blood flow, hormone production, and absorption and utilization of essential nutrients, aloe may be one of the most effective treatment aids in the course of improving the body's ability to function with diabetes.

High Blood Pressure

Like diabetes and obesity, high blood pressure was once thought of as a condition that occurred only in adults. However this condition is becoming more and more prevalent in children, striking adolescents and children as young as five. With the growing statistics that show no sign of high blood pressure being controlled or minimized, attention is now being focused on the causes and prevention. Knowing the harmful effects of sugar, fats, and additives in processed foods on the cardiovascular system's components and functioning, the blame is being placed on the diets of these young people. Through a diet of whole foods, free of chemicals, dyes, preservatives, and added sugars and fats, a child can thrive without the concern of high blood pressure, and aloe can help in every step of prevention and treatment.

Rich in vitamins, minerals, and antioxidants, aloe vera is not only able to help reduce the incidence of high blood pressure through balancing nutrient deficiencies and improving the cardiovascular system's functioning, but also by helping to maintain blood health in a number of ways. Triglycerides, blood sugar levels, and harmful plaque-depositing formations found in the blood all combine to produce harmful effects within the cardiovascular system, raising the risk of developing high blood pressure.

With aloe vera's ability to regulate blood sugar levels, reduce the amount of bad cholesterol (LDL) while raising good cholesterol levels (HDL), and effectively cleanse the blood of fatty components that clog and complicate the cardiovascular system's functioning, aloe is one of the most beneficial additions to a child's diet. Further improving a child's ability to combat high blood pressure, aloe vera enables absorption and use of specific nutrients like calcium, zinc, and magnesium that directly promote the blood's health as well as the nerve system's and cardiovascular system's functioning in which the blood plays major roles. Through a diet of nutrient-dense, natural foods that contribute essential nutrients, free of processing and additives, a child's blood and body benefit immensely in a number of ways, one being a lower risk of high blood pressure. The recommended daily dose of ½–1 tablespoon of aloe vera can provide a child with blood-pressure benefits, while teens may require a gradually increased daily dose between 1–2 tablespoons of aloe vera for improved blood pressure benefits.

Fatigue

Without a doubt, your diet is directly related to your energy level. With a quality diet, the nutrients the body needs are ever present, allowing for the bones, muscles, and brain to be engaged on demand without issue. With a poor diet lacking in essential nutrients, the result can be chronic fatigue that limits a child's ability and desire to engage in physical activity. While this may seem like an insignificant situation that is isolated to only particular points of deficiency in a child's life, the results are not so time specific.

When the body is deficient in essential nutrients, the fatigue that results can be felt over the course of days, weeks, and even months. Insufficient supplies of the nutrients needed leads to underuse and dysfunction of every system and function in the body, and the body's physical manifestation of these deficiencies and dysfunctions is reduced energy levels. With little energy and less activity resulting, the body can begin to experience atrophy, further contributing to bouts of fatigue and inactivity, and the cycle continues on and on until the deficiencies are corrected.

Through its own provision of vitamins, minerals, amino acids, and powerful phytochemicals that act as antioxidants, aloe vera can help deliver much-needed nutrients. Added to a diet of whole foods that contribute the bulk of macronutrients and micronutrients needed for a child to thrive, aloe can improve energy levels and reduce the incidence of fatigue. Each and every system throughout the body is able to function properly through the support of nutrients, enzymes, and phytochemicals that aloe provides— whether the improvements are a result of improved immunity, ample supplies of nutrients, improved nutrient absorption, improved enzymatic activity, or reduced carcinogenic activity within cells. The benefits to the body's energy levels can be seen through improved attention and focus, higher energy levels, improved metabolic functioning, and increased ability of the bones and muscles to perform basic functions needed for activity and recovery.

Sleep

Sleep is absolutely essential for optimal health. Without sufficient sleep, both in terms of amount and quality, the mental and physical health of a child can be adversely affected. With dysfunction wreaking havoc on everything from digestion, mood, focus, behavior, and metabolism, a child suffering from inadequate sleep can live a life of turmoil. With simple adjustments and the implementation of healthy habits, any child can reap the benefits of restful nights' sleep that allow the body and mind to readjust, replenish, and rejuvenate, helping any child rediscover the fun of childhood every day. Good sleep habits during childhood can continue well throughout adulthood as well.

Nutritional Needs and Functions

The nutrition a child receives from his meals throughout the day can have a major impact on the sleep cycle. With a routine of regularly set meals and snacks that provide the body with adequate energy supplies throughout the day, the body is able to taper off its responses to stimuli as a child nears bedtime. With the last meal being provided at least one hour before a child's bedtime, digestion is able to take place long before the child drifts off to sleep. The normal activity of digestion (and any adverse reactions that could lead to "tummy troubles") occur well before the body begins to rest and relax; without the interference of digestive processes or problems, the body is able to fall asleep and stay asleep, reaping the benefits of the restorative nutrients consumed in the last meal of the day.

Physical Activity and Energy Levels

With physical activity, the body is able to use its stores of energy, and it depends on the body's natural sleep processes as a time of repairing the body and brain and preparing energy stores for the following day. With energy expended, the body and mind are able to sleep more restfully while the "behind-the-scenes" breakdown and replenishment of nutrients used by the body's organs and systems is able to take place. Through the natural sleep cycles of a child, the levels of energy are regulated, making energy available for use the next time it is required. Without adequate sleep, the muscles, bones, and brain begin to conserve energy, minimizing energy levels available for energy output. With adequate sleep, though, the body is able to thrive, restoring a balance of nutrients that provide the fuel for the workings of the entire body's organs, systems, and processes.

Mental Functioning, Mood, and Behavior

It's no secret that the quality of one's sleep can positively or negatively affect behavior and mood. With adequate sleep, brain functioning, cognition, focus, and behavior improve, and the behavior of well-rested children is directly reflected in their mood, school performance, and relationships with peers, authorities, and family. This creates situations in which a child is able to reap the benefits of positive feedback that contribute to a cycle of better performance, more positive feedback, and so on.

Conversely, a lack of sleep can produce erratic moods, mental fatigue, drastically impaired focus and attention, and may even result in outbursts and behavioral upsets. These symptoms not only affect a child's environment, but can also create internal anxiety and self-esteem issues. Poor sleep habits can create a negative feedback cycle, resulting from poor behavior and performance, begetting negative feedback that only further perpetuates the cycle. Being studied more and more every year, the connection between sleep and depressive disorders, anxiety, and attention disorders produce the same results: Sleep is absolutely essential for the mental health and optimal functioning of the developing brain in children.

How Aloe Can Help

Aloe vera can help with digestion, regulate blood sugar levels, and reduce the incidence of digestive troubles through its provision of phytochemicals, but it can also improve a youngster's quality of sleep through its amino acids like tryptophan that help produce the sleep-related hormones that allow the brain and body to relax and move through the appropriate stages of sleep as intended. With the use of aloe vera, not only are the physical stores of essential nutrients supported through the unique provision of aloe's own vitamins, minerals, and phytochemicals, but the benefits to sleep throughout the bedtime routine can be impressive as well.

In children, the process of "winding down" at bedtime can be riddled with fluctuations in mood, excitement, and energy, leading to a challenging time that is anything but conducive for sleep. Aloe vera's calming amino acids like tryptophan can calm the body and brain, and its blood sugar stabilizing benefits can help your child achieve better sleep easily, safely, and naturally. In terms of mood and behavior in children, aloe vera can also provide positive results with the support of the mental processes and the production of essential hormones that help children benefit from better cognitive functioning, stable mood, and less depressive disorders.

Recipes

Great Green Berry Blast

This great-tasting smoothie is packed with vitamins, minerals, amino acids, enzymes, and antioxidants to improve and protect a child's overall health.

INGREDIENTS | SERVES 4

¼ cup aloe vera juice

2 cups organic apple juice

½ cup chopped spinach

½ cup blueberries

½ medium apple, peeled and cored

Combine all ingredients in a blender. Blend until smooth.

Sweet Strawberry Shake

*Kids will love this nutrient-rich snack, which supports the functioning
of the entire body's processes, especially the brain!*

INGREDIENTS | SERVES 4

¼ cup aloe vera juice

2 cups unsweetened vanilla almond milk

1 cup frozen strawberries

2 tablespoons ground flaxseed

Combine all ingredients in a blender. Blend until smooth.

Cough-Calming Cooler

You can help your child overcome a cough or calm respiratory dysfunction without over-the-counter cough syrups. This natural remedy contains anthocyanins and antioxidants that contribute to the respiratory system's functioning, along with honey's naturally occurring antibacterial and antimicrobial properties.

INGREDIENTS | SERVES 2

¼ cup aloe vera juice

2 cups brewed chamomile tea, chilled

½ cup frozen blueberries

½ cup frozen blackberries

1 tablespoon pure organic honey

1 teaspoon ground cinnamon

Combine all ingredients in a blender. Blend until smooth.

Sweet Dreams Tea

By minimizing exposure to stressful situations, allowing for a period of "winding down" time before bed, and focusing on nutrition, you can help your child sleep better. This deliciously sweet smoothie provides natural antioxidants and calming phytochemicals that contribute to healthy sleep so your child can rest easy and sleep more deeply.

INGREDIENTS | SERVES 2

⅛ cup aloe vera juice

1 cup brewed chamomile tea, chilled

½ medium banana, peeled and frozen

½ tablespoon pure organic honey

Combine all ingredients in a blender. Blend until smooth.

Mock Chocolate Milk

Almond milk and dates combine to create a delicious smooth taste similar to chocolate milk. With essential nutrients galore, and without any of the unhealthy ingredients, this is one "chocolate milk" recipe that parents can feel good about and kids can love!

INGREDIENTS | SERVES 4

¼ cup aloe vera juice

2 cups unsweetened almond milk

4 large dates, pitted

Combine all ingredients in a blender. Blend until smooth.

CHAPTER 13

Aloe Vera and Women

Regardless of age, relationship status, or interests, women are connected through common experiences. Fluctuations, phases, and experiences in life that are specific to women should be addressed and treated with a different view than those used to treat "the average person." Through years of research and studies, women have more answers now than ever about how they can improve the quality of their lives. With fitness, nutrition, reduced stress, restful sleep, better focus, and improved immunity, women are able to enjoy longer, healthier, happier lives. And, of course, aloe can help!

Women's Health

Women's health is not only different from men's, but requires specific attention at various points throughout life as well. As women age, the processes their bodies go through are very different, changing drastically even from one year to the next. With normal phases like monthly menstruation, times of pregnancy, menopause, and aging in general, the systems of a woman's body have specific needs. Since so many systems contribute to the overall health and well-being of a woman, it is easier to understand women's health by identifying the significance of the systems, the importance of their functioning, and how to optimize each in order to achieve better health.

Cardiovascular System

The importance of the cardiovascular system to a woman's health cannot be emphasized enough. This system and its components are directly responsible for supporting the functioning of every organ, system, and process of the body. While pregnant, a woman's cardiovascular system also supports the health and well-being of her unborn child. Throughout a woman's life, the health of her blood, proper functioning of her heart, and ability of her cardiovascular system to adequately supply her body and brain with blood, oxygen, hormones, and nutrients can dictate the health and quality of life she enjoys.

ALERT

While most people think that the symptoms of heart disease are associated with the chest or area of the heart, this leading killer of both men and women is more commonly associated with symptoms such as nausea, jaw pain, and shoulder pain. If you suffer from any of these symptoms frequently, contact your physician for a consultation in reference to possible heart disease assessments.

Skin Health

While men are more likely to succumb to skin-related illnesses caused by the sun, women are still at risk. Years ago, this issue was considered purely aesthetic, based mostly on the connection between the sun and wrinkles. Today, we know the devastating consequences of skin cancers, and it is absolutely essential for every woman to safeguard her skin, not only for cancer prevention, but for the maintenance of an immune system that can be adversely affected by illnesses and diseases related to or resulting from neglect in the area of skin care.

Digestive System

The digestive system of a woman is not only responsible for digestion, but plays a major role in infections of the reproductive system. Yeast infections, urinary tract infections, and a number of common health issues in women are directly associated with the diet and a woman's production of healthy bacteria in the gut. Safeguarding this system with a balanced diet that provides the body with essential nutrients helps protect against illness and disease, while also ensuring that uncomfortable conditions don't wreak havoc on daily life.

Endocrine System

The natural hormone estrogen that allows for the female body to function and maintain a feminine appearance (breast and hip development) can contribute to deadly conditions like cancers when not regulated properly. Too much or too little of any hormone can lead to mental and physical dysfunction, which is precisely why the endocrine system, the hormones it controls, and the support a woman can provide to it must be a point of focus when the goal is optimal health.

FACT

Family history of breast cancer may not be the only indicator of a woman's risk for developing breast cancer. While mutations of inherited genes play a part in the development of the cancer that is second only to lung cancer in women's cancer deaths, other risk factors such as early menstruation (prior to the age of twelve), late menopause (after the age of fifty), and not having any children throughout one's childbearing ages have been determined as risk factors as well.

Skeletal System

Knowing that calcium deficiency contributes to the millions of cases of osteoporosis around the globe, every woman should recognize the importance of supplying the skeletal system with essential nutrients. This framework that provides the body with support in many more ways than just structure can improve or degrade the quality of a woman's life. With stores of nutrients, multiple functions that support the body in everyday life, and its contributions to the processes of countless systems, the skeletal system should always be cared for and supported through nutrition, activity, and protection.

ALERT

Osteoporosis, the deterioration of bone density over time, strikes both men and women. Of the 44 million Americans who develop osteoporosis every year, though, a startling 68 percent are women. By focusing on a diet rich in vitamin A and calcium, allowing for 10–15 minutes of sun exposure daily, and engaging in regular strength training activities for thirty minutes at least three times per week, women can reduce their chances of developing osteoporosis.

Respiratory System

Chronic conditions that attack the respiratory system can result in life-altering limitations and even death. With every system throughout the body dependent upon the oxygen that is inhaled through the lungs and processed through the respiratory system, taking care of this system is beneficial to the entire body as a whole. With direct effects on the brain and cardiovascular system, disease prevention, stroke prevention, and the maintenance of physical and mental well-being, care for the respiratory system is an absolute must in women's health.

Immune System

From the common cold to specific cancers, the immune system acts as the body's line of defense in maintaining overall health in a woman.

Impacting every function and process in the body, the immune system is one of the most important areas of focus in maintaining a woman's health. Through simple steps that can help safeguard immunity and improve the performance and functioning of the immune system, a woman can remain strong and sickness-free not only on a daily basis, but well throughout life.

Fitness

"A body in motion stays in motion" has never rang more true than in today's society. With more and more evidence supporting this statement, we now know that fitness and regular exercise play a major role in the length of life and quality of life. For women, engaging in physical fitness routines on a regular basis not only helps maintain motor control, but can also affect every aspect of life, from mental stability and hormone balance to increased energy levels and improved sexual performance. This all-encompassing aspect of health is not isolated to the hour at the gym or the Monday-morning yoga class, but, instead, an empowering life-improving regime that has a positive impact on self, health, and life.

Physical Functioning

Physical fitness has its most obvious results in the physical functioning of the body. With cardiovascular exercise, strength training, flexibility, and stretching, a woman engages her body in activities that promote the health and well-being of every system and function in her body. With the skeletal system and muscular systems being utilized to perform and support the movements of physical fitness, it's no surprise that physical activity directly promotes the strength and stability of the bones and muscles. By routinely engaging in fitness routines, the female body also benefits from improved cardiovascular health and optimal cardiovascular system functioning, improved digestion, and even better brain functioning and nerve cell functioning. All these areas combine to benefit the body as a whole.

Aloe vera can help any woman maintain a physical fitness routine in many ways. Between its topical uses that can help relieve muscle soreness produced by inflammation and restore essential nutrients to the bloodstream, and its internal uses that provide support to the existing and strengthening bones and muscles, aloe can be used as an effective element that can improve the results of a physical fitness routine. By helping the cardiovascular system function properly with a cleaner composition of blood, helping the bones maintain strength, and optimizing the nutrient absorption and use that directly promotes the muscle gained through physical fitness, aloe vera can offer the support needed in maintaining a body that can engage in motion and stay in motion.

Hormones and Happiness

The "feel-good" hormones that are released when one engages in physical activity are not the only hormonal benefit of exercise. The exciting and rejuvenating feelings that are felt after exercise are only a portion of the hormonal results that benefit the body as a whole. The glands and organs that are responsible for producing and processing hormones reap immediate and long-term benefits from exercise, helping these areas better regulate the precise hormones that positively affect mood, energy level, regular menstruation, internal body temperature regulation, and metabolism. Even insulin and blood sugar levels can be optimized through the hormonal benefits of exercise, helping to regulate mood, hunger, and energy even more. The increased blood flow during and following exercise helps ensure each and every system and organ receives adequate supplies of blood, oxygen, and essential nutrients, further supporting health throughout the body.

ALERT

A startling 12 million women suffer from some sort of depressive disorder every year. Whether the depression is a result of a biological imbalance or life event, many psychiatrists recommend that women battling depression reach out for connections. Through the development of relationships among family and friends, at work, or within the community, many women report feeling less depressed.

With proper functioning of hormone-producing systems and organs, and the regularity that is restored to all areas of the body as a result, the reports of overall happiness by those who engage in regular exercise are, not surprisingly, higher than those who do not. One's self-esteem, self-worth, energy levels, positivity, and self-reported feelings of success and achievement have all been shown to improve, and these "feelings" are further supported by the hormone levels, brain activity, and physical results that are positively affected by exercise. This cyclic reaction continues and improves, impacting areas of life that may seem unrelated; digestion, sexual desire and stamina, motivation, concentration, and even the quality of your skin, nails, and hair can all benefit from physical fitness.

How Aloe Can Help

Packed with essential nutrients that help the body process, use, and stabilize hormone levels throughout the body and in a number of various functions, aloe vera is able to support the systems and processes that stabilize mood and promote happiness. With plentiful B vitamins that directly promote the functioning within the brain and between the brain and body, aloe vera can help your brain's processing of the feel-good hormones that are produced with exercise, and it can also help the physiological processes that are engaged in bouts of physical fitness. The bones, muscles, and complex systems that all take part in the physical fitness are even further supported not only by the nutrients provided by aloe, but also by the added benefit of improved absorption of these essential nutrients caused by the phytochemicals contained within aloe.

Aloe has shown to be a remarkable addition to the areas of health like physical fitness and activity in a number of ways. It helps improve energy levels, maintaining optimal metabolic functioning and supporting the muscles, bones, and organs that are involved in the processes that are engaged with physical activity. Aloe vera provides the nutrients needed for activity while improving the cardiovascular system's delivery of those nutrients, supporting the skeletal and muscular system's absorption and utilization of essential nutrients, and providing the nervous system with the support it needs in order to communicate effectively between the brain and body. The cardiovascular, skeletal, muscular, and nervous systems all reap benefits from aloe and its components, allowing women to continue in their physical fitness routines and experience the plentiful benefits of those routines.

Nutrition

The female body's need for nutrients is as unique as the life phase she is in at any given moment. Whether the phase is puberty, pregnancy, menopause, or any area of life in between, the need for specific vitamins, minerals, and essential nutrients is different, but crucial. The iron needs in times of menstruation are far different from the needs for calcium during menopause, the need for B vitamins is far more crucial for fertility than at any other point in life, and so on. Knowing the key nutrients that can help optimize the functioning of the female body at any specific point can help in the maintenance of health and happiness throughout a long life of many different phases.

Menstruation

The blood lost in menstruation is a natural monthly process that allows for life to change and be created. While this natural process has occurred since the beginning of time, the information available to women today can help relieve associated discomforts while restoring and replenishing the essential stores of nutrients lost in the process. Knowing that iron stores are depleted with the blood lost in the menstrual flow, it is essential to focus on iron supplementation through food and supplements. In addition to iron, an increased focus on B vitamins can not only help reduce the incidence of premenstrual syndrome, but can also minimize the fluctuations in mood, lack of attention or focus, and loss of energy due to the menstrual process. Aloe vera not only provides these essential nutrients, but also helps promote the absorption and utilization of these vitamins and minerals and supports the systems that utilize the nutrients.

Fertility

Anyone who has tried to become pregnant knows that waiting for the positive pregnancy test result can be excruciating. That stress has actually been proven to lessen the chances of becoming pregnant, adding stress to the list of factors that can postpone conception. With a focus on nutrition during the times of preparing for pregnancy, a woman can reduce her stress and optimize her fertility, greatly improving her chances of conception. Whole foods rich in B vitamins help maintain positive balances in mood, reducing stress that can interfere with fertility, while also improving the stores of the essential B vitamin folate needed at conception and throughout the course of pregnancy. Iron, magnesium, and calcium are among the top fertility-improving nutrients that fend off deficiencies that can inhibit conception. Each of these nutrients, along with the powerful phytochemicals that aloe also contains, combines to protect against illnesses and deficiencies that can plague fertility in childbearing years.

Pregnancy

Pregnancy is a 40-week experience that is far different from any other part of life. With every passing week, the needs fluctuate depending upon the development taking place. From the point of conception, the nutrient needs of a fetus create demands on the body of the expectant mom; these sudden requirements can result in fluctuations within the mom's hormones, systems, and bodily functions that can lead to fatigue, morning sickness, and lack of focus. Replenishing stores of vital nutrients like iron, calcium, magnesium, B vitamins, and zinc not only help provide the growing baby with the essentials needed for proper development, but also help support the health of the mom-to-be.

ALERT

It is important to note that because of the restrictions and limitations placed on studies of pregnant women, the statistics surrounding aloe vera use during pregnancy are minimal. You should consult with your doctor before supplementing your diet in any way while pregnant.

Aloe vera provides the crucial nutrients needed for pregnant women and their babies, it can improve the absorption of certain nutrients (especially the B vitamins, calcium, iron, and zinc), and it may help minimize the uncomfortable side effects of pregnancy like nausea and constipation. Because of this, supplementation of aloe vera during pregnancy is a topic that is receiving growing attention from the medical community. With the added benefits of improving immunity and protecting cells from disastrous changes, aloe vera's phytochemicals may prove to be vital additions to the perfect prenatal diet. As with all aspects of pregnancy, it is absolutely imperative that a pregnant patient considering adding aloe vera to her daily routine consult her physician prior to doing so.

Menopause

"The change" that occurs in every woman is viewed as an uncomfortable and undesirable aspect of life by women around the world. Often characterized by mood swings, restless nights, and hot flashes, it's no wonder that this natural transition is notorious. With a focus on nutrition, though, many women are able to move through menopause with minimal physical and mental discomfort. Consuming a diet rich in iron, calcium, and B vitamins can directly support the needs of the body as it transitions through menopause, minimizing the deficiencies that result in the fluctuations of mood, internal temperature, and energy levels. The body's use of essential nutrients that can quickly become depleted as the hormonal and physical changes of menopause take place can be supported with a diet focused on nutrient-dense foods, and supplementation of nutrient-rich additions like aloe vera.

Packed with vitamins, minerals, and aloe-specific phytochemicals, aloe vera is able to support the natural physical changes that take place in menopause without undesirable side effects that can result from over-the-counter and prescription aids. Because aloe helps improve the brain's functioning and helps regulate mood with B vitamins, supports energy levels and helps maintain proper metabolic functioning that can better regulate internal temperatures with iron, and provides phytochemicals that directly promote sleep for those restless nights, aloe is growing in popularity as a menopause treatment. Further supporting the proper diet with its phytochemicals that improve absorption and utilization of the much-needed vitamins and minerals, aloe vera may be the perfect supplement for prevention and relief during this time.

Optimizing Any Age

With the ebbs and flows of physical needs throughout life, listening to your body can provide the most accurate information about what your body requires. While the nutrient needs of a twenty-year-old are different from that of a sixty-year-old, the physical manifestations of nutrient deficiencies can be extremely similar. By focusing on a diet of whole, nutrient-dense foods and limiting the sugary, sodium-laden processed foods, the benefits to the female body can be nothing short of miraculous . . . regardless of age.

Ensuring that the needs of immunity-boosting vitamin C, fatigue-fighting iron, bone-building calcium, and mood-enhancing B vitamins are adequately supplied can be difficult when the stresses and schedules of daily life leave time and focus limited. Supplementing with aloe vera can help, though. With its ability to help the body function optimally, reduce the risk of deficiencies and their physical manifestations, and directly promote the systems that help women maintain the energy, focus, metabolism, and overall health they need to be their best at all times, aloe can support all women of all ages by ensuring the body has what it needs to do what it needs when it needs to do it!

Stress

Children, careers, relationships, and life experiences give meaning and significance to life. However the responsibilities of supporting and maintaining them can sometimes lead to stress. Stress and anxiety, while seemingly harmful to everyday life, can actually be positive. Identifying sources of stress can prove to be beneficial by illuminating situations that need attention.

Uncontrolled stress and anxiety can wreak havoc on your physical, mental, and emotional processes, leading to negative drains on your health and quality of life. Meditation, journaling, regular exercise, and proper nutrition can all serve as helpful stress-reduction areas of focus that provide the body's physical and mental processes with support in times of need. Through simple steps that care for your physical and mental well-being, you can minimize stress and reap benefits that improve your health and foster a balance within yourself and throughout your life.

With stress playing a major role in the development of serious illnesses and conditions that can severely affect life, stress is an area that should be addressed in every woman's life. Excessive stress has been shown to contribute to high blood pressure, cardiovascular disease, weight gain, weight loss, reduced mental functioning, fatigue, and may even hinder nutrient absorption. While this natural element of life serves its purpose to promote healthy awareness, allowing stress to become an uncontrollable element of daily life can result in disaster. With a number of proven methods that can help alleviate stress and reduce the physical and mental impact it can have, women can take control of their stress and regain balance in their lives. Surprisingly, aloe can help in the area of stress by contributing nutrients and phytochemicals that support various body systems that play a role in stress, both directly and indirectly.

Deep-Thinking Exercises

Through thought exercises like meditation and journaling, it can be easier to identify situations, emotions, and experiences that are causing stress, helping to bring about an awareness that (in and of itself) can provide relief of stress. With an increased awareness of the sources that create stress, it can be easier to either avoid or resolve the areas of life that lead to stress. Whether the clarity results from a few quiet minutes of deep thought, pages in a journal that help thoughts that would never be spoken to be expressed, or a simple conversation with a trusted friend that gives insight and unexpected ideas on a situation, deep-thinking exercises can prove helpful in reducing stress.

Exercise

Through regular exercise, the brain's functioning and body's hormone levels can be optimized to provide the brain and body with what it needs to fend off stress and the negative hormones that result. Cortisol is the fight-or-flight hormone that increases in times of stress. Naturally intended to provide the body with immediate energy needed to protect itself, cortisol levels can remain heightened when stress and anxiety are consistent, which leads to a cycle of stress, hormone fluctuations, more stress, more hormone fluctuations, etc. With regular exercise, the body and brain are able to communicate more efficiently about the hormones produced, and the hormones related to stress are maintained at optimal levels.

Nutrition

With adequate supplies of the nutrients needed by the body, a quality diet can actually help reduce stress in a number of ways. Plentiful B vitamins have shown to directly promote brain functioning and assist in the balance of mood; iron, magnesium, and zinc help provide neurotransmitters with essential building blocks used for the creation and maintenance of the nerve cells that communicate between body and brain, helping to reduce mood swings and improve attention and focus; and the amino acids that play a role in metabolism functioning and hormone production help regulate everything from weight, energy levels, and thought processes. Focusing on a diet that provides these essentials can help in any stress-reduction plan.

How Aloe Can Help Stress

In every area of stress reduction, aloe can provide support that can improve the benefits to the brain and body, and assist in restoring the balance that results when stress is controlled. With better brain functioning, the deep-thinking exercises that play a role in stressing less can be more effective. Aloe vera provides plentiful vitamins and minerals that directly promote brain function and communication between the brain and body. Aloe vera use also promotes blood flow and optimized cardiovascular system functioning. An added benefit of the improved cardiovascular functioning is a lower incidence of high blood pressure, which is commonly seen in women with high stress levels.

With the ability to improve hormonal levels associated with mood, energy, and metabolism, aloe vera is also able to help reduce the incidence of mood fluctuations while improving energy levels and metabolic functioning; through these areas, aloe vera is able to support the physical requirements and benefits that revolve around the physical fitness aspect of stress reduction. In terms of nutrition, the use of aloe vera helps promote nutrient absorption and utilization that directly promotes the systems that work in the process of reducing stress. Aloe vera can help support each and every aspect of stress reduction, improving the results and increasing the benefits to help any woman achieve the balance she needs for a healthier, happier life.

Immunity

Without question, any discussion about health must include a focus on immunity and illness prevention. The immune system and all the body's support systems that help maintain its proper functioning protect a woman from illnesses and diseases. By improving the functioning of the immune system, the very aspects of health become stronger, and lead to a cycle of improved performance of every system, further supporting the immune system, and perpetuating a self-reliant system that results in more energy, better sleep, improved sex drive, proper metabolic functioning, and (of course) fewer incidences of illnesses and disease.

As with all aspects of health, the immune system benefits or suffers as a result of a number of factors. Even lifestyle factors that seem to be completely unrelated to immunity can have an impact on another system on which the immune system relies; the complexity of the inner workings of the body are, arguably, best illustrated with an understanding of the functioning of the immune system, which relies on and affects every aspect of the body and its health in one way or another.

Because of the immune system's dependence on other systems of the body, it is important to care for the body as a whole, rather than specifically focusing on improving the immune system. Taking into consideration that the cardiovascular system, skeletal system, digestive system, and nervous system play intricate roles in the processes that support the immune system's functioning, any woman can see the importance of total-body care when focusing on improving immunity. Taking control of the lifestyle factors that help or harm the body can help in maintaining optimal system functioning, directly supporting the immune system and improving the efficiency of a woman's immunity.

In every area of health, aloe can help in a variety of ways that either directly or indirectly promote the best functioning of a particular system or process. Through nutrients provided, improved absorption of the essentials, phytochemicals that target infectious compounds, and antioxidants that act to support cell health, aloe vera is a remarkable addition to any woman's life in terms of immunity support.

Digestion

Without proper functioning of the digestive system, every area of the body suffers. The digestive system is not only responsible for the processing of food, but also provides the body with most of its immunity support. The digestive system is able to purge harmful bacteria, viruses, and microbes that attack any part of the body, ridding these illness-causing agents from the body; this is why vomiting and diarrhea are two of the most common symptoms that result from illness. Through the aloe-specific phytochemicals that act in the digestive system as support for the removal of harmful microbes, and the restorative properties that help the digestive system and its organs recover from illnesses, aloe is able to improve the immunity-promoting power of the digestive system naturally.

Sleep

Sleep is important for immunity; it is an essential restful recovery time the body needs in order to replenish stores of nutrients and revive systems that have been engaged for hours while awake. With minimal sleep or reduced sleep quality, the effects on immunity can be severe, resulting in more frequent bouts of illness and a higher chance of developing disease. Through regular consumption of 1 tablespoon of aloe vera approximately one hour before bed, a woman can experience better quality sleep with the added bonus of a more efficient immune system.

Activity

With regular exercise and activity, the demands on the cardiovascular system directly promote the proper functioning of every system in the body. By promoting improved blood flow, adequate hormone production, improved sleep, proper digestion, and better brain functioning, exercise not only improves overall quality of life, but can also act synergistically to support the immune system. With the improved functioning of the body, and the positive effects this optimal functioning has on each and every system in the body, the demands on the immune system are also decreased, allowing the immune system to attack illness- and disease-causing agents when they develop.

Nutrition

With adequate amounts of the essential nutrients that are required by the body, every cell, organ, and system is able to function as intended. Vitamins A, C, and E work together with powerful minerals like zinc and magnesium (just to name two) as antioxidants that support the immune system's "seek and destroy" process of protecting cells from harmful elements that can cause dangerous changes within cells. Adding to the cell protection benefits of nutrients, specific phytochemicals have been known to improve the quality of the blood by cleansing harmful agents that could result in illness and disease, making natural, whole foods a superior source of nutrition that serves as protection.

How Aloe Vera Can Help Immunity

By not only providing vitamins A, C, and E, but also improving the body's ability to absorb these essential vitamins, aloe vera can help directly support the immune system's functioning. Adding aloe to your health routine can help ensure that the essentials are available and utilized properly. These vitamins also act as powerful antioxidants that improve the body's ability to prevent harmful changes at a cellular level. When these powerful vitamins combine with aloe's phytochemicals, which not only act as antioxidants but also provide protection against bacteria, viruses, fungi, and microbes, the protection and prevention of the immune system and all the body's systems can be seen in reduced illnesses.

Recipes

Cranberry Cleanser

Cranberries contain natural proanthocyanins that help protect against adhesive bacteria that can cling to the walls of the urinary tract, which helps prevent urinary tract infections. With the added benefit of vitamin C and powerful antioxidants that help improve immunity, this delicious smoothie allows you to sip your way to better health!

INGREDIENTS | SERVES 4

¼ cup aloe vera juice

2 cups brewed green tea, chilled

½ cup frozen cranberries

1 tablespoon organic maple syrup

Combine all ingredients in a blender. Blend until smooth.

Creamy Banana Smoothie

This smoothie contains ample amounts of calcium for bone health and probiotics, which ensures the digestive tract is free of harmful microbes that can interfere with the body's ability to absorb and use the essential mineral.

INGREDIENTS | SERVES 2

¼ cup aloe vera juice
1 cup unsweetened vanilla almond milk
1 cup plain Greek yogurt
1 medium banana, peeled and frozen

Combine all ingredients in a blender. Blend until smooth.

Banana-Flaxseed Smoothie

The average woman's diet is lacking in omega fatty acids, which have been shown to help regulate the natural hormones in the body. This smoothie provides ample amounts of omegas, along with vitamins, minerals, and flavor!

INGREDIENTS | SERVES 2

¼ cup aloe vera juice

2 cups unsweetened almond flax milk

½ cup hemp seeds

¼ cup flaxseed

½ cup chopped walnuts

1 medium banana, frozen and peeled

Combine all ingredients in a blender. Blend until smooth.

Nutty Pumpkin Smoothie

Magnesium and manganese found in pumpkin flesh and seeds can help reduce bloating, boost your mood, and improve the quality of your sleep. If you suffer from PMS, try this delicious smoothie to minimize symptoms.

INGREDIENTS | SERVES 2

¼ cup raw unsalted pumpkin seeds

¼ cup aloe vera juice

1 cup pumpkin purée

2 cups unsweetened vanilla almond milk

½ teaspoon ground cloves

½ teaspoon ground cinnamon

1 tablespoon organic maple syrup

1. Combine pumpkin seeds and aloe vera in a blender, and blend until seeds are emulsified.

2. Add remaining ingredients, and blend until all ingredients are thoroughly combined.

CHAPTER 14

Aloe Vera for Men

Men have specific needs in terms of improving health and quality of life. Providing protection against the illnesses and diseases that are common among men, along with the promotion of the health throughout the body's systems, aloe vera has been shown to be a powerful addition to the life of any man. By taking control of the lifestyle factors that contribute to their health and well-being, and using aloe to support those healthy choices, men can experience better health and a better quality of life, naturally.

Men's Health

With different hormones, different physical composition, and different systematic activities, the needs of men's bodies are very different when compared with that of women and children. These drastic differences contribute to the unique needs of men in terms of physical activity, nutrition, sexual health, mental well-being, and beyond. For specific areas of concern, men are also encouraged to focus on improving and maintaining the health of the following systems.

Cardiovascular System

The American Heart Association estimates that one out of every three men currently has some form of cardiovascular disease. Cardiovascular disease can lead to heart attacks, heart conditions, strokes, and heart disease. The American Heart Association stresses the importance of overall health in reducing the incidence of cardiovascular-related illnesses and diseases with a focus on physical activity, a clean diet of nutrient-dense foods, and reduced stress.

ALERT

The American Heart Association estimates that one out of every three men will develop some form of heart disease in their lifetime. In order to maintain a lifestyle that minimizes the chances of developing cardiovascular disease and stroke, refraining from smoking, minimizing drinking, eliminating stress, consuming a heart-healthy diet, and engaging in regular physical activity can all help to promote heart health and minimize your risk.

Skin Health

Men are more than twice as likely as women to develop some form of skin cancer in their lifetime. With this deadly condition developing quickly, and its ability to metastasize to other areas of the body in a short period of time, it is crucial for men to maintain annual screenings for skin health. Prevention and treatment of skin conditions can prevent disastrous complications that result from cancerous changes within the skin's cells; early detection of these changes can be the difference between life and death.

Digestive System

Home to the functions that are responsible for the processing of food, absorption of nutrients, and the delivery of the nutrients required by the entire body and its systems, the digestive system plays a role in almost every aspect of men's health. In the digestive system, the process of ridding the body of its waste is an area of concern because colorectal cancer is one of the most prevalent types of cancer in men. With the digestive system playing such an important role in the prevention of illness and the promotion of health, and also being the site of possible cancerous complications, the health of this system should be a focus in every man's life.

Endocrine System

Testosterone is responsible for an astounding number of functions in a man's body, from energy and stamina to muscle maintenance and bone health. The endocrine system is responsible for the production of testosterone and is directed by the hypothalamus and pituitary gland, both located in the brain. With optimal functioning of the endocrine system, a man experiences adequate sperm production, high levels of energy and stamina, and more efficient muscle and bone health maintenance. Supporting the endocrine system with exercise, a balanced diet, and an avoidance of harmful factors like smoking and alcohol consumption is a must for improving and maintaining men's health.

Skeletal System

Just as calcium is important for women in the maintenance of bone health, men require ample nutrients that support the skeletal system and its processes. While discussions of osteoporosis more commonly focus on women, men are susceptible to the deterioration of the bones. By optimizing the factors that contribute to the health of the skeletal system, men can not only improve their overall health, but also reduce the incidence of injury and illness.

Respiratory System

With lung cancer and respiratory diseases on the rise, a program focused on the improvement of men's health must include the respiratory system. While most people only think of the respiratory system as being responsible for breathing, this system also plays an intricate part in the systematic functioning and processes throughout the body. By safeguarding respiratory health, each and every system within the body is able to function more efficiently, while reducing the chances of developing illness and disease in the area.

Immune System

The immune system is the body's line of defense against illnesses and diseases that range from mild to severe. Even responsible for the maintenance of cellular health, the immune system plays a role in the processes involved in every function of the body. Reducing the incidence of contracting colds and flus and minimizing the possibility of dysfunctions and the development of disease, a focus on maintaining a healthy immune system benefits the body in countless ways.

Fitness

Physical activity helps the body maintain proper functioning of the muscles and bones while also improving the body's health. Not just affecting the physical aspects of health, physical activity can also assist in the maintenance of brain functioning and the hormones related to happiness. Balance among the body's systems is essential for any health promotion program, and regular physical activity can create balance and improvement of the health of both body and mind.

Physical Functioning

With regular exercise, the body is able to benefit from improved delivery of the essential nutrients needed throughout the body. While the most notable improvements take place in the cardiovascular system, the benefits of exercise are quickly reflected throughout the body. The improvement in blood pressure, blood health, and the functioning of the heart, blood vessels, and arteries directly promotes overall health by providing blood flow to all the body's organs and systems.

FACT

In an original research article published in *Environmental Toxicology and Pharmacology* in December 2014, the effects of topical aloe vera in minimizing the appearance of wrinkles on the skin were explored, leading researchers to conclude that regular use of aloe vera can deliver nutrients and collagen-building proteins directly to the skin, helping to minimize the appearance of fine lines and wrinkles.

The improved nutrient delivery that results from better cardiovascular performance impacts the quality of the bones and muscles immensely. With adequate supplies of calcium and amino acids being delivered, the bones remain strong and dense and the muscles are able to maintain mass and respond to the demands of physical activity. The brain also benefits from exercise by receiving improved blood flow and responding to the physical demands with ample amounts of hormones. These hormones not only improve performance, but also contribute to the maintenance of optimal blood sugar and fat levels.

Hormones and Happiness

In every human body, the levels of hormones directly affect health and happiness. With excessive amounts of any hormone, extreme highs and lows can result in fluctuations of mood, focus, energy, metabolism, and even anxiety. Conversely, hormones in low levels can result in dysfunctions of the body's organs and systems, wreaking havoc on everyday life and contributing to the development of illnesses and disease.

From sexual well-being and stamina, high energy levels, and optimized metabolic functioning to a balanced positive perception and mood, hormones play a major role in the healthy man's life. With each aspect of health being utilized in one form or another in work, sex, sleep, and play, the hormonal balance within a man is essential. Regular physical activity results in improved balance of testosterone, serotonin, and a number of other essential hormones in the body's physical and mental processes.

ALERT

The Centers for Disease Control and Prevention reports that twice as many men suffer from alcohol-related illnesses when compared with women. The startling fact is that excessive alcohol abuse can increase the risks of developing serious illnesses and diseases like cancers of the mouth, throat, esophagus, and liver, as well as depression, and a higher risk of suicide.

With the increased hormone production and regulation taking place during and after exercise, the results increase the probability of engaging in future exercise and reaping the feel-good benefits, perpetuating a cycle of exercise and benefits that continues to contribute to overall health every day for the rest of a man's life.

How Aloe Can Help Fitness

Aloe's unique blend of vitamins, minerals, and phytochemicals support the physical activity in men by improving the systems that are engaged during exercise and contributing to the processes that improve health as a result. With the amino acids necessary to support muscle health, aloe vera not only contributes to the muscular system's functioning, but also in the preparation of the muscles for future work, enabling them to engage in activity, and reducing the downtime needed for muscle repair after activity. The bones that lend the support structure for the movements and mobility needed for exercise depend on the intake and stores of essential vitamins and minerals; aloe vera not only supplies nutrients needed by the bones, but can also improve the ability of bones to absorb and utilize the nutrients consumed in the diet.

In terms of hormones, the brain's response to physical activity is improved with a number of effects that aloe has on the body. Aloe helps clean blood move more efficiently throughout the brain and body, optimizes functioning of the nerve cells throughout the brain and body, and provides a more efficient supply of nutrients for the production and utilization of hormones in a variety of systems, all of which help the brain receive messages and respond accordingly more efficiently.

Nutrition

Nutrition plays a major role in the health of men. Helping to promote the activities needed to stay healthy, support the processes that maintain overall health, and provide the building blocks necessary for every organ, tissue, and function within the body, nutrients can make or break a healthy lifestyle. The nutrients you supply your body for use in every function are imperative to preventing illness and living a long and healthy life!

Vitamins

A diet packed with essential vitamins can improve a man's health and vitality immensely. Deficiencies of any of the essential vitamins can lead to physical and emotional hardships, but there are a handful of vital vitamins that have direct effects on the abilities men depend on each and every day. Between cognitive functioning, physical strength, and balancing mood, the following vitamins can correct imbalances, restore health, and rejuvenate the body's systems:

- **B vitamins:** The B vitamins play a crucial part in the brain, nervous system, and throughout the body. B vitamins help improve cardiovascular health and reduce the risk of cardiovascular issues like high blood pressure, irregular heartbeat, and high cholesterol content in the blood. Additionally B vitamins support the functioning of muscles by aiding in the contractions required for movement, and support metabolism and energy levels that are needed for everyday activities as well as exercise-specific actions. With aloe vera providing every one of the B vitamins, it's no surprise that regular aloe vera use can not only help support these areas of health, but also add even more support through its provision of the essential minerals like zinc needed to utilize the vitamins efficiently.

FACT

- **Vitamin C:** Acting to support the immune system, vitamin C also provides support to the cardiovascular system by ridding the blood of carcinogens and harmful agents that can lead to complications, illnesses, and disease. With ample amounts of vitamin C, men can prevent the incidence of cardiovascular diseases, heart attacks, and even strokes. Aloe vera helps in the absorption of vitamin C and further supports the immune system's protection against illness and disease by contributing its own doses of vitamin C and powerful antioxidants that contribute to a healthy immunity.
- **Vitamin D:** Commonly referred to as the sunshine vitamin, vitamin D is an essential vitamin that the body produces after exposure to sunlight. While this essential nutrient can also be found in cow's milk and eggs, the most efficient way to obtain vitamin D is through brief bouts of sun exposure. Because of the elevated risk of skin cancer in men, aloe actually helps the body obtain vitamin D from sunlight safely by protecting the skin's cells from harmful UVA and UVB rays that can create cancerous changes, allowing for the brief sun exposure needed with less risk.

Minerals

The activity in the body that is supported through adequate mineral intake is nothing short of astounding. The cells of the brain, skeleton, muscles, and even immune system all depend upon specific minerals to function properly. Minerals are an area of nutrition that should be given a great deal of attention in order to optimize performance and maintain overall health.

- **Zinc:** Required by the brain in order to produce essential neurotransmitters used in the processes of communicating between the brain and body, zinc is an essential mineral that does double duty by supporting the immune system functioning as well. Aloe vera not only provides zinc, but also improves the body's use of the mineral by supporting the functioning of the systems that contribute to the processing, storage, and utilization of the mineral.
- **Calcium:** Even though women are considered to fall victim to osteoporosis more often, men can also suffer from bone density issues that result from inadequate calcium supplies and stores. With insufficient supplies of calcium through the diet, the body turns to stores of calcium in bones and teeth, leading to osteoporosis and even dental health issues. Through its own stores of calcium, aloe vera can improve the skeletal system through supplementation in addition to its assistance of delivery of the nutrient through its support of the cardiovascular system's functioning.
- **Selenium:** This little-known mineral is responsible for a lot of physical and mental processes that can improve overall health and well-being. Working to support the brain's activity, selenium also contributes to the development of sperm, helping to regulate sperm production and improve sexual performance. Aloe vera is one of the few natural sources of this mineral that also provides support for its absorption and utilization by promoting the health of the very systems that are responsible for its delivery and use: the endocrine and cardiovascular systems.

Phytochemicals

The naturally occurring chemicals found within plant-based foods can help protect and promote a man's health and well-being in a number of astounding ways. Phytochemicals not only promote proper system functioning and protect against illness, but can also provide support to specific organs and processes that are significant in the maintenance of men's overall health and well-being.

Through the direct promotion of hormone production, phytochemicals can improve everything from cognitive to sexual functioning. With powerful antioxidants that act as scavengers of free radicals and cancer-causing agents, phytochemicals are also able to safeguard a man's health and improve the immune system's protection against illness and disease. Also improving the body's ability to absorb and utilize nutrients consumed in the diet, phytochemicals can assist in the skeletal, muscular, endocrine, and nervous systems' functioning, the most likely areas to suffer as a result of deficiencies.

Mental Health

Men are more likely to develop depression and depressive disorders than any other part of the population. Stress, sleep, physical changes, diet, and physical activity all contribute to a balanced state of mental health and well-being, but these areas are the most likely to be neglected by men. In order to maintain mental health and avoid depressive difficulties, it is absolutely imperative for men to focus on improving these areas of health. With simple steps, and the use of aloe vera, these areas of life can be improved and maintained.

Stress

Stress is an everyday part of life. Stress indicates a disruption in the norm, whether it be with emotions, situations, or people, stress is your body's natural way of increasing awareness and attacking a problem or issue in order to restore balance. Stress can help you become more aware of your internal and external needs that should be addressed in order to restore the body and mind to a state of normalcy. Without addressing the issues that cause stress, though, a continued upset can occur that wreaks havoc on the body and mind. Within the brain, stress triggers the release of hormones that directly affect the rest of the body's systems.

Everything from heart rate and blood pressure to digestion and energy levels function in ways that are intended to support the body's reactions to stress, but when stress continues for prolonged periods of time, the dysfunction of the body's systems continues as well. Within the brain, the hormones that are causing the upset in the body's systems take away from the necessary normal functions of the brain, leading to confusion, inability to focus, and sever cognitive dysfunction. By identifying the issues that lead to stress and handling the issues in whatever way is most appropriate, stress levels can be efficiently decreased, restoring health and balance.

Sleep

The natural sleep rhythms allow for the brain and body to restore and replenish for optimal functioning following sleep. The interruption of normal sleep patterns can cause major difficulties in the area of mental health. Sleep is necessary to allow every system to refuel, and without the recommended 6–8 hours of sleep, the entire body begins to feel the effects.

Synergistically, the systems and functions throughout the body rely on one another, and when one system is adversely affected, the rest suffer both short-term and long-term. The effects are felt after just one restless night, with less energy, less strength, interrupted focus, and a less balanced mood. Each of the factors that contribute to overall mental and physical health are affected, which can lead to a cycle that consists of more nights of less sleep, more mental and physical dysfunction, and the results become more consistent, perpetuating the cycle further.

With inadequate sleep, the brain and body communication that is needed for decision-making, reflexes, focus, and awareness is interrupted and slowed. Even within the brain, inadequate sleep can cause reduced hormone production and utilization, creating dysfunction throughout the body and an upset within the levels of biochemicals associated with depression. Having a higher incidence of depression, men should concentrate on the quality of their sleep, making an effort to achieve regular seven to eight hour intervals of uninterrupted, restful periods of shut-eye.

Diet

Knowing that the nutrients needed by the body serve a purpose in not just one, but many, processes, it's no surprise that the effects of a quality or deplorable diet can be seen and felt in the mental aspects of health. Nutrition affects the hormones directly associated with balanced mood, energy levels, and metabolic functioning. Without consuming the proper balance of carbohydrates, proteins, and fats, as well as the vitamins, minerals, and essential nutrients, a man's cognitive functioning and focus can be negatively affected.

When a man's diet includes the elements necessary for the brain and body to function as intended and communicate properly, the chances of developing mood disorders, anxiety, and depressive dysfunctions is reduced immensely, making a quality diet focused on whole, nutrient-dense foods a matter of mental health and overall quality of life!

Physical Activity

The brain and body respond to physical activity in ways that directly promote mental health and well-being. When the body is engaged in physical exercise, and for hours and even days afterward, the cardiovascular, respiratory, endocrine, digestive, and immune systems function differently. The respiratory system takes in more oxygen, the cardiovascular system delivers more blood and oxygen throughout the body, and the brain releases feel-good hormones that send messages to the body that initiate higher energy levels, better sleep patterns, improved digestion, and a more balanced mood. All these factors directly contribute to the improved mental functioning and overall mental health of a man.

Sexual Health

Erectile dysfunction is one of the most negative aspects of a man's health because it acts as a catalyst and also a result. With optimal sexual health, a man is able to experience arousal, engage in sex, and benefit from the natural hormonal fluctuations that result from climax; this process, and the natural hormone fluctuations that take place in the brain and body as a result, lead to feelings of relief, less stress, and an overall sensation of enhanced mood and positive self-esteem.

When the normal process is interrupted, the brain and body suffer from hormonal imbalance, increased stress, negative self-talk, and reduced self-esteem, all of which contribute to the increased likelihood that future sexual performance will be interrupted. This cycle can wreak havoc on the mental health of a man, resulting in mood swings, lack of energy, interrupted cognitive functioning, anxiety, and depression.

In order to maintain overall health and well-being, men should consider the factors that contribute to optimal sexual performance that include all the aspects of mental health: stress, sleep, diet, and physical activity. By caring for each of these areas of health, most men can ensure that sexual health is maintained well throughout life, leading to improved mental health and quality of life.

How Aloe Can Help Mental Health

Aloe vera can improve the reduction of stress, both physically and mentally. By providing ample amounts of every B vitamin, aloe vera can support the brain's functioning and cognitive reasoning abilities, helping to reduce the incidence of stress before it even occurs. Through its provision of vitamins and minerals that directly support the cardiovascular system, aloe vera can also help reduce blood pressure that heightens as a result of stress. Even in terms of digestion, the effects of aloe vera can be beneficial in times of stress; the powerful phytochemicals in aloe vera act to support healthy digestion and prevent common digestive issues such as constipation that are normally experienced in times of stress.

Immunity

Quickly and easily, any man's health can be adversely affected by infection, illness, or disease, and for this reason, the care for the body's immunity, and each of its supporting systems, should be an area of focus. With an increased awareness of how lifestyle factors and aloe vera can work hand in hand to provide the body with an element of protection against contracting illness and disease, any man can take proactive steps that not only improve overall health, but also safeguard that health.

With a focus on maintaining the health of all the body's systems through lifestyle choices like nutrition, physical activity, proper sleep, reduced stress, etc., a man can easily provide the care needed to support the body's immune system. Aloe vera cannot only act to provide protection against harmful infectious agents, but can also improve the body's ability to remove the infectious properties and the cells that have already been damaged as a result.

Recipes

Peach-Banana Smoothie

*L-arginine is an amino acid that has been shown to improve the blood flow
to the precise parts of the body in need when erectile dysfunction and excessive dryness
occur. This smoothie's ingredients not only provide L-arginine, but also promote
sex drive with omega and B vitamins that help improve mood and brain functioning.*

INGREDIENTS | SERVES 2

¼ cup aloe vera juice

2 cups unsweetened vanilla almond milk

½ cup dry rolled oats

2 tablespoons ground flaxseed

1 medium banana, peeled and frozen

½ medium peach, peeled and pitted

Combine all ingredients in a blender. Blend until smooth.

Pomegranate Tea

With rich anthocyanins and specialized phytochemicals that help promote the health of the prostate, pomegranate can help reduce the risk of prostate cancer.

INGREDIENTS | SERVES 2

¼ cup aloe vera juice
1 cup brewed green tea, chilled
1 cup organic pomegranate juice
1 tablespoon organic maple syrup

Combine all ingredients in a blender. Blend until smooth.

Green Protein Smoothie

Complex carbohydrates, protein, and omegas can boost the brain and body with improved functioning, better health, and protection against commonly experienced age-related degeneration of the bones, muscles, and brain.

INGREDIENTS | SERVES 2

¼ cup aloe vera juice

2 cups brewed green tea, chilled

½ cup chopped spinach

½ cup chopped kale

½ medium apple, peeled and cored

½ medium pear, peeled and cored

¼ cup ground flaxseed

Combine all ingredients in a blender. Blend until smooth.

Plum Smoothie

Here's a tasty way to stay regular and feel great! With the added benefit of vitamins, minerals, and antioxidants that promote health and well-being, this delicious drink is a knockout win for any man who wants to live better!

INGREDIENTS | SERVES 2

¼ cup aloe vera juice

2 cups unsweetened vanilla almond milk

6 dried plums, pitted

1 medium banana, peeled and frozen

1 teaspoon ground cinnamon

Combine all ingredients in a blender. Blend until smooth.

Superman Coffee

This morning cup of coffee is not your average cup of Joe. Bursting with health-promoting and health-protecting nutrients, this coffee recipe also provides caffeine for energy, and medium-chain fatty acids that promote brain functioning. For better health, energy, focus, and immunity, look no further than this delicious morning pick-me-up!

INGREDIENTS | SERVES 2

¼ cup aloe vera juice
12 ounces hot brewed caffeinated coffee
2 tablespoons organic coconut oil
1 teaspoon ground cinnamon
⅛ teaspoon ground cayenne pepper

1. Combine all ingredients in a blender with the opening adjusted to allow heat to be released.

2. Blend until ingredients are thoroughly combined and coffee looks light brown and frothy.

Blueberry-Almond Smoothie

Loaded with L-arginine, zinc, omegas, and calcium, this delicious smoothie provides the ingredients for improving the health of the systems that contribute to testosterone production.

INGREDIENTS | SERVES 2

¼ cup aloe vera juice
1 cup unsweetened almond milk
1 cup plain Greek yogurt
½ medium banana, peeled and frozen
½ cup frozen blueberries
1 tablespoon ground flaxseed

Combine all ingredients in a blender. Blend until smooth.

CHAPTER 15

Aloe Vera Safety and Concerns

While the benefits of aloe vera have been well documented and are supported by research studies, there are some concerns about its safety. As with all things, natural and manmade, the safety of applying something to the body or ingesting it can raise concerns about possible adverse side effects. Recently, scientists and researchers have provided the public with important information about aloe and its safety, restoring the temporarily marked reputation of aloe and reviving the faith of its loyal consumers.

A Scar on the Healing Plant

In 2002, the safety of aloe came into the spotlight . . . and it was not a positive light. With reports of stomach pain, diarrhea, and even cancerous developments being attributed to the use of aloe, consumers became concerned about the aloe plant's safety and the health risks associated with aloe-containing products. In the following years, research studies were performed to identify the cause of reported issues, and the single study that shook the aloe-loving world was released in 2004.

ALERT

The World Health Organization estimates that 2.2 million people suffer from adverse drug reactions annually. Taking medications properly and as instructed is thought to be safe, but even the most commonly pre-scribed pharmaceutical medications can lead to adverse reactions.

This study and its statistics, which were presented by a reputable govern-ing agency (the Food and Drug Administration, responsible for protecting consumers' health) evoked fear and skepticism about this natural healing plant that had been used in medicinal treatments for thousands of years. The backlash of this report resulted in doubts about aloe's safety and led to a reduction in purchasing, production, and use of aloe.

Aloe and the FDA

The Food and Drug Administration (FDA) is responsible for protecting the public health by assuring the safety, efficacy, and security of human and veterinary drugs, biological products, medical devices, our nation's food supply, cosmetics, and products that emit radiation. While the FDA is responsible for maintaining the safety of the foods and medications that are consumed by the American public, there are no standards or regulations used to determine the safety of herbs or supplements. For years, though, aloe was one of the main ingredients of laxatives provided to consumers in over-the-counter treatments and prescription medications intended to relieve constipation. In 2002, the FDA pulled all aloe-containing laxative treatments, citing concerns over the risks that could result from use of aloe products. In the years that followed, extensive research was performed on aloe and its components to determine whether there were real risks posed by aloe consumption.

FACT

Like all other regulated industries, the use of botanicals in the manufacturing of foods, drugs, and cosmetics is overseen by a government agency, the Food and Drug Administration (FDA), to ensure the safety of consumers. Through the implementation of rigorous standards that demand proven safety trials and extensive testing of botanicals, the FDA regulates all "natural" products.

With the growing concern about aloe and its safety, the FDA chose to release the findings of a study that was performed to determine the health risks associated with aloe consumption. The January edition of the journal *Toxicological Sciences* featured the data provided by FDA scientists showing that lab rats who had consumed aloe vera over the course of two years suffered from tumors and cancerous growths; the scientists concluded that aloe was no longer to be considered safe for human consumption, deducing that the consumption of aloe vera would produce the same effects in humans as it had in the laboratory animals. While these findings were soon to be exposed as flawed, the damage had already been done, and the great debate about aloe and its safety was ignited.

The Healing of Aloe's Reputation

The response to the FDA's release of the findings and conclusions resulting from the aloe study were catastrophic, creating fear and doubt among the very people who had embraced aloe as a natural alternative to harsh, synthetic treatments. The medical community became wary of the plant and its safety, and were quickly separated into two groups: those who refused to administer or recommend aloe until research proved it to be safe, and those who adamantly believed the findings of the FDA study to be false.

Regardless of which side of the issue one took, the obvious question everyone was wondering was, "How could a plant that had been used for thousands of years suddenly be harmful instead of helpful?" The

International Aloe Science Council (IASC) took on the challenge of answering that exact question, and presented the FDA and the public with a collection of research, studies, statistics, and findings from years of in-depth experimentation and observation of aloe and its components, providing hard evidence about the real risks and benefits that result from its use.

Through dedication and determination, the IASC was able to refute the findings of the FDA aloe study and restore the reputation of aloe and its benefits, bringing the miraculous healing plant (and its benefits) back to the aloe lovers who had trusted it.

Is Aloe Safe?

While some people assume that because something is "natural," it is safe, this is hardly the case. There are a number of natural elements like plants, animals, and gases that are unsafe, or even deadly. While natural elements have a more closely related biological element shared with humans, something being natural does not deem it safe by any means.

Aloe is one of the natural gifts of the world that is able to provide amazing benefits, but it can also contain specific elements that should be avoided. While the harm and side effects that can result from handling or ingesting these elements is minimal, it is beneficial to any community to have certain parameters and guidelines in place to protect manufacturers and consumers from harm that can be caused through the improper production of aloe vera or treatments using aloe vera.

FACT

In an original research study, "Beneficial effects of Aloe vera in treatment of diabetes: Comparative in vivo and in vitro studies," researchers studied the effectiveness of aloe vera on improving the body's ability to produce and process insulin. Having determined that aloe vera is an effective natural treatment for diabetes in returning the body's blood sugar levels and insulin-producing ability to normal, aloe vera is being researched in clinical trials as a possible treatment for the disease.

Recognizing this fact, the International Aloe Science Council was created, and it is this council that tries to educate people on the uses and side effects of aloe. The IASC is a nonprofit organization that has created standards to which aloe products are held in order to maintain the safety of the products in which aloe is used.

Aloe's Aloin Content

In regards to the FDA findings, the question of whether it was the aloe content that had contributed to severe stomach issues still remained. The IASC and a number of scientists took on the responsibility of identifying the specific element of aloe that could be responsible for such discomfort (if there indeed was one). They discovered that an aloe compound, aloin, could produce stomach irritation, and should be minimized or avoided completely in order to prevent discomfort, diarrhea, etc.

While the initial reaction was that this conclusion would again cause consumers to be wary of aloe, the IASC insisted that the finding was a positive one. The discovery enabled the IASC to test aloe and aloe-containing products, and ensure that none of the IASC-certified products would include agitating levels of aloin, making IASC-certified aloe products safer than ever before.

Having determined through numerous studies that the source of stomach issues related to aloe is due to aloin, or aloe latex, the IASC developed standards that required aloe products to contain a maximum allowable amount of aloin in products made available to the public. Through this new testing, manufacturers of aloe and aloe-containing products have been able to provide an assurance of safety to consumers, minimizing the possible side effects that can result from aloe use.

The IASC seal of approval can be found on multiple products containing aloe, and has been recognized by the FDA as an important certification that consumers should look for when choosing aloe products.

Aloe and Cancers

Attacking the second issue posed by the FDA's findings in lab rats, the IASC joined forces with the International Agency for Research on Cancer (IARC) to determine the contributing factors that could pose health risks related to carcinogenic activity from aloe consumption. Not only was the IASC able to produce several published studies that found no carcinogenic activity in lab rats who had been provided aloe vera, but they also determined through experimental research that unpurified whole-leaf aloe that had not been decolorized was the harmful form that could possibly contain toxic elements. While the amount of aloe (unpurified and not decolorized) that would have to be consumed to produce cancerous changes would far exceed any normal consumer's regular use, the IASC and IARC moved to reduce the carcinogenic compounds from aloe products. Having developed tests for these toxic elements as well, the IASC is able to maintain the safety and efficacy of aloe products made available to consumers.

Defending the reputation of aloe through proven findings, while also instituting measures used to deem products as safe for consumption, the IASC has saved the reputation of aloe and restored consumers' faith in the product that has, and will continue to, bring about benefits that improve lives around the world.

Harmful Combinations

While aloe vera has the ability to contribute unique properties to the body, enhance the effectiveness of naturally occurring nutrients, and improve the body's ability to absorb and utilize nutrients, there are concerns about certain interactions. People who suffer from specific illnesses and diseases can experience difficulties when care is not taken to ensure safety.

Because aloe vera has been proven to produce effects on the blood and the body's functions, the main concerns about aloe risks pertain to people who are taking supplements or medications, and undergoing treatments with which the benefits of aloe can interfere. There are specific combinations in which aloe vera should never be included, and knowing these dangerous combinations is the most effective way to safeguard one's health and avoid complications.

Diabetes

Diabetes patients are commonly prescribed insulin and blood-sugar regulating medications that are intended to maintain a steady level of blood glucose in the blood stream. Effective as a treatment, insulin is injected into the bloodstream, lowering the blood sugar levels to a safe range.

Aloe vera has shown in numerous studies to positively benefit those who suffer from diabetes by naturally restoring a balance of blood sugar. Because of its effectiveness in reducing blood sugar levels, aloe vera is commonly suggested for use by prediabetics or diabetics. However, aloe vera should never be used with insulin or other blood-glucose medications. By using both aloe vera and blood-sugar-regulating medication, blood sugar levels can be drastically reduced, resulting in conditions that are just as dangerous as those experienced when blood sugar levels are too high.

Potassium Deficiency

Many prescription medications have the side effect of reducing the potassium levels in patients. Studies have shown that aloe provides the benefit of maintaining adequate levels of potassium when taken alone, but increases the effects of medications that produce the potassium-lowering side effect. In order to avoid the risk of developing serious potassium deficiencies, it is recommended that a patient discuss the possibility of potassium-related side effects with his physician prior to combining aloe with medications of any kind.

Diuretics

The result of taking a diuretic is reduced water content in the body. Many people take diuretics in order to reduce bloating, but the impact on the body can be severe. With the loss of essential water stores, the body can become dehydrated and experience deficiencies in the levels of minerals and electrolytes. While aloe is able to provide essential nutrients and electrolytes, studies have shown that aloe maximizes the effects of diuretics, resulting in extreme water loss and reduced blood sugar levels.

Laxatives

Not surprisingly, the aloe that was once used for laxative purposes can increase the effects of stimulant laxatives. Even though the components of aloe responsible for purgative reactions have been minimized or removed completely, studies have shown that aloe is able to intensify the effects of stimulant laxatives; therefore, aloe and laxatives should not be combined.

Who Shouldn't Use Aloe?

When it comes to people who have specific conditions, aloe vera hasn't been studied to lengths that allow for safe recommendations on its usage. Because of the restrictions and concerns that relate to testing supplementation on developing children, women who are pregnant, and people with disorders that could possibly be adversely affected or aggravated as a result of experimentation with supplements, the information available on the safety of aloe is simply not available.

There have been reports of allergic reactions to the topical applications of aloe vera and products containing aloe. With millions of people using aloe vera topically and experiencing benefits from the plant's liquid and gel, the percentage of those who experience adverse reactions of the skin is extremely small. Because the possibility of experiencing a rash, irritation, or allergic reaction does exist, the most widely accepted recommendation for those with sensitive skin is to spot test aloe vera on a small area of the skin before applying the liquid or gel to the intended area of treatment; if no irritation occurs within 10–15 minutes following the application, the aloe vera can be applied to larger areas of skin.

Providing vitamins, nutrients, amino acids, and a variety of unique phytochemicals that have shown to produce amazing results in terms of health issues, aloe is regarded as one of the most beneficial supplements available. With this information, many people have used aloe vera by their own choosing, experiencing results that have improved conditions of all kinds.

While there are warnings about aloe vera use designed to protect people against the possible risk factors, the possibility of experiencing adverse reactions solely from aloe vera use are minimal. By speaking with a physician, doing research on the risk factors that could pose complications from aloe vera use with specific conditions, and focusing on your body's responses to the use of aloe vera, you can determine if adding aloe vera to your daily routine is safe for you.

APPENDIX A:

Online Resources

Aloe Medical Group International

The Aloe Medical Group International is a homeopathic and naturopathic education group that promotes the use of aloe to heal a variety of conditions.

www.aloe-medical-group.com

Diabetes.co.uk: Aloe Vera and Diabetes

This article covers research into the use of aloe vera to improve blood glucose levels.

www.diabetes.co.uk/natural-therapies/aloe-vera.html

International Aloe Science Council

The International Aloe Science Council (IASC) is a leading authoritative voice on aloe, aloe products, and consumer safety. The IASC is regarded as the most reputable source of certification for aloe product manufacturers. Their website provides consumers with a wealth of information on the history, harvesting, and production of aloe vera around the world.

www.iasc.org

Lily of the Desert

Lily of the Desert is a reputable aloe vera manufacturer with tons of aloe products. Their website also serves as a great source of information on aloe and its effects on health.

www.lilyofthedesert.com

Natural Medicine Journal: "Aloe Vera Research Review"

This article is an overview of many research trials that have been done to study the effects of aloe vera on several health issues.

http://naturalmedicinejournal.com/journal/2012-09/aloe-vera-gel-research-review

Prevention: "10 Things You Can Do with Aloe Vera"

This article includes tips for creating aloe-vera-based face wash, hand sanitizer, and other DIY health and beauty products.

www.prevention.com/beauty/beauty/10-things-you-can-do-aloe-vera

Pub Med: "The Effect of an Aloe Polymannose Multinutrient Complex on Cognitive and Immune Functioning in Alzheimer's Disease"

Here's a link to a study on aloe as a possible treatment to improve functioning in Alzheimer's patients.

www.ncbi.nlm.nih.gov/pubmed/22976077

Pub Med: "Effect of Aloe Vera Gel to Healing of Burn Wound: A Clinical and Histologic Study"

This is a link to an article about a clinical study involving aloe vera as a topical treatment method for burns. This study compared the effects of aloe vera versus a non-aloe treatment method, and found evidence that aloe heals burns effectively.

www.ncbi.nlm.nih.gov/pubmed/7561562

University of Maryland Medical Center: Complementary and Alternative Medicine Guide

This page offers information on the use of aloe vera for skin conditions, constipation, diabetes, and dental health.

http://umm.edu/health/medical/altmed/herb/aloe

Scientific Studies Proving Benefits of Aloe Vera

Immunity

"Isolation and characterization of novel protein with anti-fungal and anti-inflammatory properties from Aloe vera leaf gel" (Original Research Article) *International Journal of Biological Macromolecules*, Volume 48, Issue 1, 1 January 2011, Pages 38–43. Swagata Das, Biswajit Mishra, Kamaldeep Gill, Md. Saquib Ashraf, Abhay Kumar Singh, Mou Sinha, Sujata Sharma, Immaculata Xess, Krishna Dalal, Tej Pal Singh, Sharmistha Dey

"Mass spectrometry characterization of an *Aloe vera* mannan presenting immunostimulatory activity" (Original Research Article) *Carbohydrate Polymers*, Volume 90, Issue 1, 1 September 2012, Pages 229–236. Joana Simões, Fernando M. Nunes, Pedro Domingues, Manuel A. Coimbra, M. Rosário Domingues

"Antioxidant properties and PC12 cell protective effects of APS-1, a polysaccharide from Aloe vera var. chinensis" (Original Research Article) *Life Sciences*, Volume 78, Issue 6, 2 January 2006, Pages 622–630. Jun H. Wu, Chen Xu, Cheng Y. Shan, Ren X. Tan

"*In vitro* and *in vivo* antioxidant activities of polysaccharide purified from aloe vera (*Aloe barbadensis*) gel" (Original Research Article) *Carbohydrate Polymers*, Volume 99, 2 January 2014, Pages 365-371. Min-Cheol Kang, Seo Young Kim, Yoon Taek Kim, Eun-A. Kim, Seung-Hong Lee, Seok-Chon Ko, W.A.J.P. Wijesinghe, Kalpa W. Samarakoon, Young-Sun Kim, Jin Hun Cho, Hyeang-Su Jang, You-Jin Jeon.

Skin

"Anticedants and natural prevention of environmental toxicants induced accelerated aging of skin" (Original Research Article) *Environmental Toxicology and Pharmacology*, In Press, Accepted Manuscript, Available online 3 December 2014. Tanuja Yadav, Shivangi Mishra, Shefali Das, Shikha Aggarwal, Vibha Rani

"Preliminary evaluation: The effects of Aloe ferox Miller and Aloe arborescens Miller on wound healing" (Original Research Article) *Journal of Ethnopharmacology*, Volume 120, Issue 2, 20 November 2008, Pages 181–189. Yimei Jia, Guodong Zhao, Jicheng Jia

"Skin permeation enhancement potential of Aloe Vera and a proposed mechanism of action based upon size exclusion and pull effect" (Original Research Article) *International Journal of Pharmaceutics*, Volume 333, Issues 1–2, 21 March 2007, Pages 10–16. L. Cole, C. Heard

"Aloe vera for preventing radiation-induced skin reactions: a systematic literature review" (Original Research Article) *Clinical Oncology*, Volume 17, Issue 6, September 2005, Pages 478–484. J. Richardson, J.E. Smith, M. McIntyre, R. Thomas, K. Pilkington

Brain

"Susceptibility of hippocampus and cerebral cortex to oxidative damage in streptozotocin treated mice: prevention by extracts of Withania somnifera and Aloe vera," *Journal of Clinical Neuroscience*, Volume 11, Issue 4, May 2004, Pages 397–402. M.S Parihar, Madhulika Chaudhary, Rajani Shetty, Taruna Hemnani

Cancer

"Isolation and identification of a phenolic antioxidant from Aloe barbadensis" (Original Research Article) *Free Radical Biology and Medicine*, Volume 28, Issue 2, 15 January 2000, Pages 261–265. Ki Young Lee, Susan T. Weintraub, Byung Pal Yu

"Anticancer potential of emodin" (Review Article) *BioMedicine*, Volume 2, Issue 3, September 2012, Pages 108–116. Shu-Chun Hsu, Jing-Gung Chung

"Vitamin c and aloe vera supplementation protects from chemical hepatocarcinogenesis in the rat" (Original Research Article) *Nutrition*, Volume 14, Issues 11–12, November–December 1998, Pages 846–852. Nor Aripin Shamaan, Khalid Abdul Kadir, Asmah Rahmat, Wan Zurinah Wan Ngah

"Chemomodulatory action of Aloe vera on the profiles of enzymes associated with carcinogen metabolism and antioxidant status regulation in mice" (Original Research Article) *Phytomedicine*, Volume 7, Issue 3, June 2000, Pages 209–219. Rana P. Singh, S. Dhanalakshmi, A. Ramesha Rao

"Aloe vera for preventing radiation-induced skin reactions: a systematic literature review" (Original Research Article) *Clinical Oncology*, Volume 17, Issue 6, September 2005, Pages 478–484. J. Richardson, J.E. Smith, M. McIntyre, R. Thomas, K. Pilkington

Diabetes

"Beneficial effects of Aloe vera in treatment of diabetes: Comparative in vivo and in vitro studies" (Original Research Article) *Bulletin of Faculty of Pharmacy*, Cairo University, Volume 51, Issue 1, June 2013, Pages 7–11. Amira Mourad Hussein Abo-Youssef, Basim Anwar Shehata Messiha

"Antidiabetic activity of Aloe vera L. juice. I. Clinical trial in new cases of diabetes mellitus" (Original Research Article) *Phytomedicine*, Volume 3, Issue 3, November 1996, Pages 241–243. S. Yongchaiyudha, V. Rungpitarangsi, N. Bunyapraphatsara, O. Chokechaijaroenporn

Metabolism

"Metabolic effects of aloe vera gel complex in obese prediabetes and early non-treated diabetic patients: randomized controlled trial" (Original Research Article) *Nutrition*, Volume 29, Issue 9, September 2013, Pages

1110–1114. Ho-Chun Choi, Seok-Joong Kim, Ki-Young Son, Bum-Jo Oh, Be-Long Cho

Women

"Preventing skin toxicity in breast cancer patients undergoing radiotherapy with an emulsion containing hyaluronic acid, chondroitin sulfate, aloe vera, carrot oil, vitamin F and vitamin E." *Radiotherapy and Oncology*, Volume 98, Supplement 2, March 2011, Page S41. J. Pardo, M. Murcia, A. Alvarado, N. Feltes, M.L. Hernández, A.M. Pérez, J. Olivera, J. Luna, J. Vara, A. Alvarez, R. Soto, A. Biete

Safety and Effectiveness

"The aloe vera phenomenon: a review of the properties and modern uses of the leaf parenchyma gel" (Review Article) *Journal of Ethnopharmacology*, Volume 16, Issues 2–3, June 1986, Pages 117–151. Douglas Grindlay, T. Reynolds

Standard U.S./Metric Measurement Conversions

VOLUME CONVERSIONS

U.S. Volume Measure	Metric Equivalent
⅛ teaspoon	0.5 milliliter
¼ teaspoon	1 milliliter
½ teaspoon	2 milliliters
1 teaspoon	5 milliliters
½ tablespoon	7 milliliters
1 tablespoon (3 teaspoons)	15 milliliters
2 tablespoons (1 fluid ounce)	30 milliliters
¼ cup (4 tablespoons)	60 milliliters
⅓ cup	90 milliliters
½ cup (4 fluid ounces)	125 milliliters
⅔ cup	160 milliliters
¾ cup (6 fluid ounces)	180 milliliters
1 cup (16 tablespoons)	250 milliliters
1 pint (2 cups)	500 milliliters
1 quart (4 cups)	1 liter (about)

WEIGHT CONVERSIONS

U.S. Weight Measure	Metric Equivalent
½ ounce	15 grams
1 ounce	30 grams
2 ounces	60 grams
3 ounces	85 grams
¼ pound (4 ounces)	115 grams
½ pound (8 ounces)	225 grams
¾ pound (12 ounces)	340 grams
1 pound (16 ounces)	454 grams

OVEN TEMPERATURE CONVERSIONS

Degrees Fahrenheit	Degrees Celsius
200 degrees F	95 degrees C
250 degrees F	120 degrees C
275 degrees F	135 degrees C
300 degrees F	150 degrees C
325 degrees F	160 degrees C
350 degrees F	180 degrees C
375 degrees F	190 degrees C
400 degrees F	205 degrees C
425 degrees F	220 degrees C
450 degrees F	230 degrees C

BAKING PAN SIZES

American	Metric
8 x 1½ inch round baking pan	20 x 4 cm cake tin
9 x 1½ inch round baking pan	23 x 3.5 cm cake tin
11 x 7 x 1½ inch baking pan	28 x 18 x 4 cm baking tin
13 x 9 x 2 inch baking pan	30 x 20 x 5 cm baking tin
2 quart rectangular baking dish	30 x 20 x 3 cm baking tin
15 x 10 x 2 inch baking pan	30 x 25 x 2 cm baking tin (Swiss roll tin)
9 inch pie plate	22 x 4 or 23 x 4 cm pie plate
7 or 8 inch springform pan	18 or 20 cm springform or loose bottom cake tin
9 x 5 x 3 inch loaf pan	23 x 13 x 7 cm or 2 lb narrow loaf or pate tin
1½ quart casserole	1.5 liter casserole
2 quart casserole	2 liter casserole

Index

Note: Page numbers in *italics* indicate recipes. Page numbers in **bold** indicate recipe category lists.